YOGA AT WORK

Miriam Freedman was born in Czechoslovakia and emigrated to Israel after the Second World War. She studied in Jerusalem and qualified as a primary school teacher and then taught for 17 years in Israel and England in both state and private schools.

In 1967 she met Swami Visnudevananda in London who initiated her yoga training. She later studied the Iyengar method and in 1976 took her diploma with the British Wheel of Yoga. Miriam has been teaching yoga ever since, to group classes and individuals, and to seminars and workshops. In the early 1980s she studied alternative therapies, including biofeedback, autogenic training, reflexology, massage and counselling.

In 1979 she joined a meditation group whose emphasis was on silence, meditation, dream interpretation and group work. Miriam now also teaches meditation along the same lines.

Miriam is the author of *Under the Mango Tree*, a book of dreams.

Janice Hankes trained originally as a dancer and completed a degree in performing arts before embarking upon a career as a dance administrator. She worked at the Royal Academy of Dancing for five years, during which time she studied part-time for a masters degree in arts administration. She has since changed profession and is now working at Imperial College, University of London, where she is Administrator of the Graduate School of the Environment. Janice has been a yoga student of Miriam Freedman for four years and has found her yoga practice invaluable in coping with pressures of work and an upper back problem.

Also by Miriam Freedman

Under the Mango Tree

Yoga at Work

10-MINUTE YOGA WORKOUTS FOR BUSY PEOPLE

Miriam Freedman
and
Janice Hankes

ELEMENT
Shaftesbury, Dorset ● Rockport, Massachusetts
Brisbane, Queensland

In memory of Dr Frank Chandra and for G. and I.T.

Text © Miriam Freedman and Janice Hankes 1996

First published in Great Britain in 1996 by
Element Books Limited
Shaftesbury, Dorset SP7 8BP

Published in the USA in 1996 by
Element Books, Inc.
PO Box 830, Rockport, MA 01966

Published in Australia in 1996 by
Element Books Limited
for Jacaranda Wiley Limited
33 Park Road, Milton, Brisbane 4064

Reprinted June and August 1996

Cover photography by Guy Ryecart
Cover design by The Bridgewater Book Company
Design by Roger Lightfoot
Illustrations by Mike Cole
Typeset by Footnote Graphics, Warminster, Wiltshire
Printed and bound in the USA by Edwards Brothers, Inc.

British Library Cataloguing in Publication
data available

Library of Congress Cataloging in Publication
data available

ISBN 1–85230–817–6

Contents

Foreword

Yoga is essentially a system of trying to find our spiritual centre using, in a highly disciplined manner, techniques derived from activities in everyday life. These activities have been refined down to essentials, and have been intensified through special ways of performance and by ancillary techniques. In addition, the founders of yoga recognize that people are not all equal, but have different physical and mental abilities, different aptitudes, skills and temperaments. They realize that the interaction of generic, environmental and spiritual factors operate to produce more or less homogeneous, broad groups of men, each group being distinct from the other, rather than an undifferentiated uniform mass of humanity. Yogic masters have therefore prescribed different techniques for different categories of people, and so active people find karma yoga best suited to them; logical minded intellectuals prefer gyan yoga; for those who are highly emotional, the prescription is bhakti yoga; and for contemplative and intuitive types, raja yoga is the best path (see 'The Philosophy of Yoga', pp. 149–51).

There are many different associated practices, working through various sensory mechanisms. Chants affect vibration receptors, including the ears, and complicated diagrams affect consciousness through visual concentration and powerful inherent or learned associations. Movements, in the form of dances or postures done slowly and held for long periods, send signals to the brain through a variety of sensory receptors in the muscles, tendons, ligaments, joints and the inner ear.

Special forms of breathing, in addition, may alter blood chemistry and so affect awareness.

Some of these subsidiary techniques have interesting and secularly beneficial side-effects. The various postures and methods of breathing have useful physiological and medical results on the body in their own right, as well as helping the meditative experience. Some yoga centres therefore practise 'yogic therapy', which is based not only upon postures and breathing practices but also upon special dietary régimes, certain methods of cleansing different parts of the body, and various stages of relaxation, progressing through increasing degrees of autonomic control to meditation at various levels.

In England, attempts were made to gain official recognition for yoga at a time when the idea was prevalent. This is perhaps a remnant of the days of the British Raj, when it was believed that much in the Hindu way of life was based on superstition, and was therefore worthless. It was conceded that the postures might have a value in physical education, but techniques of breathing and meditation were frowned upon. This attitude has persisted for many years in the London area, although many enlightened authorities outside London long ago acceded to the demand for 'integral yoga' and run classes which cover the eight limbs of Pantajali's 'Yoga Sutra' – in theory at least.

One result of this historical legacy has been the tendency for people in the United Kingdom to regard yoga as a system of physical exercise flavoured with some simple breathing exercises. Hatha yoga has become established as a system on its own rather than as an adjuvant to raja yoga, preparing and sensitizing the mind for meditation. The emphasis here is on the body and the intellect, possibly on the emotions, but not at all on the soul.

Yoga or hatha yoga, then, has come to mean a form of physical exercise to many people. The details are based on the 'cultural' type of yogic postures which involve strong contraction of large muscle groups, combined with full stretching of various parts of the body. At the same time, many of the 'meditative' postures (which were meant to be held with the muscles relaxed) have been converted to the body-building type by holding the muscles strongly contracted whilst in the posture. A more recent development, perhaps a natural progression from the above in industrialized countries where stillness, inactivity and relaxation may be infrequently enjoyed and may later become strange or even frightening, is 'dynamic' yoga. This is where yogic postures form the basis of exercises performed with vigour or speed. These hold an attraction and benefit for certain groups of young people who are body-conscious, but can be dangerous for those who are older or unfit.

When Miriam asked me to work with her on this book, I was willing to participate because I believed it would form an essential text for people working in offices. This book describes a number of yogic postural exercises and some breathing techniques which can be done in the office during free time. Though simple, they will make more people aware of a lack of flexibility in their bodies, and will therefore call for some effort and persistence. At first, some extra motive may be necessary, such as really wanting to improve your physical condition, or to alleviate stiffness in joints after hours of sitting at a desk. Later, the feeling of well-being which follows regular performance of these exercises will become the incentive for their continuation.

Miriam and I have added our comments and some tips to most of the exercises, and have tried to alert performers to some of the mistakes commonly made, as well as to point out circumstances when certain exercises should be avoided. In all cases, any doubts should be discussed with the performer's own doctor and his/her advice should be taken in preference to any opinion expressed in this book.

DR FRANK CHANDRA

Introduction

YOGA: YOUR UNIQUE STRESS MANAGEMENT PROGRAMME

Does a day at work leave you feeling stressed out and tired? By the end of the afternoon do you ever suffer from tense shoulders, headaches, backache or eye strain? If so, keep reading because this book has been written especially for you!

You probably spend more waking hours in your workplace than you do in your own home. Yet how much thought do you give to your well-being at work? The modern work environment imposes many pressures, both physical and mental, on its workers. Display screen equipment can cause eye strain; keyboard work and other repetitive tasks carry a risk of repetitive stress injury; sitting at a desk or work station for long periods encourages postural problems and lethargy; standing for a long time can result in back problems, aching legs and feet; and air-conditioning, fluorescent lighting and lots of cups of coffee can all affect your health. Add to this the mental stress that can be caused by travelling to and from work, heavy workloads, meeting deadlines and targets and dealing with difficult people, and work can become a potential health hazard!

So how can you help yourself to survive work? This book shows you how you can adapt the system of yoga for your own work environment and help yourself tackle the everyday stresses and strains.

Since the 1960s, I have studied and worked in the field of

yoga. During this time, I have seen the benefits yoga has brought to my students, and they have repeatedly asked me to write this book. They work in a wide range of professions, and currently include lawyers, teachers, musicians, secretaries, doctors, gardeners, dancers and housewives. They have all found yoga so beneficial after an often hectic day that they do not want to have to wait for their weekly yoga class; they want exercises that they can do during the day while at work. The physical exercises given here stretch the whole body and ease stiff necks, tense shoulders, aching backs and tired legs. The breathing and relaxation exercises release tension and sooth away the stresses of the day, leaving you feeling calm and re-energized. The meditation exercises result in a feeling of inner peace and serenity.

Sounds too good to be true? Well, now it is your turn to benefit, because the good news is that we can transport part of the system of yoga into your own work environment. For many people the word 'yoga' conjures up images of people doing headstands, or tying themselves in knots in the lotus position. But there is much more to yoga than this; it is a unique system of re-balancing the body and mind that can be applied to all walks of modern life. Yoga will not only help you cope with stress at work; if practised regularly, it will change your whole outlook on life. Regular yoga practice can make you feel calmer, more in control and happier within yourself.

This manual shows you how simple hatha yoga exercises can be adapted for use in your work environment. I have selected certain exercises because they tackle the most common prob-lems experienced by workers in a wide range of professions, and I have developed and tested them on my yoga students over a period of years. The exercises do not require much space and will only take a short time to do. They include stretching, breathing, relaxation and meditation exercises.

We show you how, without even leaving your desk or work station, you can carry out simple movements that will stretch the body and ease the tension and stiffness caused by sedentary and repetitive work. The breathing, relaxation and meditation exercises form a system of stress management that can be practised throughout the day to help you to calm yourself and to re-focus and centre your thoughts.

All you need to do is set aside a few minutes each day to carry out the suggested programmes of exercises to experience the well-being that regular yoga practice brings. You can also carry out selected exercises at intervals during the day to tackle specific problems, for example the shoulder rotation exercise to ease tense shoulders or the breathing exercises to sooth your nerves. The exercises are simple and you can do most of them without drawing too much attention to yourself – but you can always get your colleagues involved and do the exercises together! It would be ideal if you could persuade your organization to set a room aside especially for this practice.

Further chapters in the book give you advice on how to improve your work environment and maximize your well-being while at work.

By practising the exercises for only a few minutes each day you will find out how the system of yoga can be your unique stress management programme at work. Stress is not inevitable. You can greatly reduce, even eliminate, it. You can help yourself to do this – the stress is yours, but so is the remedy. By reading this book, you are already taking a step in the right direction. So don't let your job sap your energy – read on and find out how to de-stress yourself at work!

Acknowledgements

The authors would like to extend thanks to the following:

Kathy Fulcher for her comments on nutrition at work; Barry McBride for photography for the line drawings; Lennie, Martin and Allison Freedman, David French, Ginger Gilmour, Sheila Griffins, June Lipka, Hilda Silver and Margaret Sampson for their general support and encouragement for this project; and to all Miriam's yoga students and teachers, past and present, who provided the inspiration for this book.

1

What is Yoga?

So what is yoga? The first image that springs to mind for many people is probably one of double-jointed people putting themselves in strange positions! But there is much more to yoga than these physical feats. We do not intend this book to be a scientific treatise on yoga; it is a practical handbook for everyday use. But before we go any further, it is important that we give you an insight into the origins of yoga and how it actually works.

Did you know that yoga is the oldest system of practical discipline known to the world? It originated thousands of years ago in India, but has only become popular in the West during the last few decades. The word yoga means union, and this is commonly interpreted as union of the body, mind and spirit. The different systems of yoga emphasize its physical, emotional and spiritual aspects: hatha and raja yoga concentrate on body and mental control; karma yoga is the yoga of action or of doing; and bhakta yoga is the yoga of devotion.

Hatha yoga is most commonly practised in the West. Through a system of physical exercises, breathing and relaxation, hatha yoga concentrates on the well-being of the body. Breath is our life force, and the breathing exercises are the most important part of hatha yoga. They cleanse the body, calm the emotions and enable you to bring your body and mind into perfect balance.

The ancient yogis, known as the Rishis, who developed this system of exercise, displayed an amazing knowledge of human beings and their anatomy. The system of exercises passed down to us today works on the body in a variety of ways; they increase the flexibility of the body, but they also work on the internal organs, the glands, the nerves and the respiratory system and so rebalance the whole body.

The Rishis were the first philosophers of India and lived close to nature. They studied man's existence in relation to nature, to plants and to animals. Many of the exercises handed down are modelled on the movements of animals and named after certain creatures; for example, the lion, the cobra and the eagle.

Yoga exercise is very different from other forms of exercise in which you might participate, for example, sport, aerobics or gym workouts. Most forms of physical exercise require a rigorous, and often competitive, use of the body to increase the heart rate and so achieve a cardiovascular workout. Such exercises often leave you feeling sweaty, exhausted and out of breath. Yoga is different. It is performed slowly and with a great awareness of your breath control. After a yoga class, you will feel invigorated, not tired. Yoga will also require you to observe how you feel, both mentally and physically, and to be aware of your personal development. The aim is not to develop muscles, but to promote suppleness, good health and the well-being of the mind, body and spirit.

Yoga is not competitive, unlike many other forms of exercise. Sport is competitive by nature, and even an aerobic class may make you feel under pressure to keep up and do as many sit-ups as possible, or keep jogging on the spot as long as everyone else! In yoga, each person's development is totally individual and you can adapt the exercises as required. For this reason yoga is popular among the elderly, with pregnant women and people with physical handicap.

The philosophy of hatha yoga treats the body as a precious resource that we have to look after carefully. Who can argue with this? We only have one body to last us a lifetime, although at one time or another we may all wish to trade it in for another model! Your body serves you and it is your responsibility to keep it in the best possible condition.

One underlying assumption of hatha yoga is that a healthy spine is essential for general good health. Good posture with the spine in perfect alignment is a starting point for yoga, and many exercises concentrate on improving the condition and suppleness of the spine.

The original system of hatha yoga comprised over 84,000 postures! Every gesture was recorded as a posture, which are often called asanas. Many of these were originally designed to be held for long periods for maximum benefit; in India some advanced practitioners have been known to stay in the head-stand for great lengths of time!

But do not panic – we do not expect you to do this! The yogis of India dedicated most of their time to meditation and performing the physical exercises. But over the years, yoga has been adapted for people like you, who cannot spare large amounts of time for their yoga practice. The number of postures has been condensed to 30–50, and in yoga classes in the West students hold a selection of exercises for shorter periods, for example, a few seconds each. In this way we can exercise the whole body in one yoga class.

If you practise yoga regularly you will feel better. Students of yoga report many beneficial effects. These include, on the physical side, increased mobility and suppleness of the body, toned and strengthened muscles, the alleviation of postural problems and, in some cases, weight loss. You will also enjoy a sense of well-being, the ability to relax quickly and effectively, a focused mind and, if you persevere, a sense of prevailing inner peace and happiness.

This is a practical guide to yoga for the workplace, but yoga also offers a deep spiritual discipline. When you practise yoga regularly you may start to experience changes in your physical, psychological and emotional states. Do not worry about this; it is quite natural. The practice of yoga over a period of time may make you start asking questions about yourself, about how you feel about certain things, about your lifestyle and your aspirations. By considering these aspects you will reach a deeper understanding of yourself: of what makes you happy and unhappy; of what you really want to get out of your life. As you begin to understand yourself more fully, you will come to appreciate life more, and be better able to cope with the stress that daily life brings.

If you want to explore further and learn more about the spiritual aspect of yoga, look for a qualified yoga teacher who will explain what is happening and how yoga has affected you in this way. Remember that although you can learn techniques and even get inspiration from books, it is by studying with a teacher that you will move further towards your goal and reach a deeper understanding of your existence. If you are interested in learning more about the complete philosophy of yoga, there is more information, and a list of further reading and details of yoga centres, at the end of the book.

There is an old saying that to achieve a balanced life we should, each day, work for eight hours, sleep for eight hours and spend eight hours on ourselves; for example, on personal development, study, spiritual awareness and spending time with our families and loved ones. Yoga can help you achieve this.

2

How Work Can Affect Your Health

The purpose of this and the following two chapters is to look at how work can affect your health and well-being. Until we know what factors at work influence us and in what way, we cannot start addressing the problems.

Work can affect you in two ways: physically and mentally. The **physical environment** in which you work – the location, furniture, equipment, heating, air conditioning etc – and the actual **physical nature** of your work, for example, sitting, standing, repetitive, strenuous or whatever, can all affect you. You can suffer directly through physical symptoms such as aches, pains, discomfort and injury, and also mentally by feeling under stress. If you suffer from mental stress over a period of time this too can manifest itself in physical problems, for example, headaches, sleeping disorders and stomach problems.

Similarly the **mental demands and pressures** of your work, for example, the deadlines, heavy workloads and people you work with, can also affect you. In the first instance you will be affected mentally; for example, you may feel under pressure, anxious, panicky, resentful or angry, but these feelings can again take the form of physical symptoms.

The following two chapters look specifically at physical and mental stress at work, and examine potential sources of stress and how they may affect you.

HOW MUCH DOES WORK AFFECT YOUR HEALTH?

Self-observation is an important part of yoga, and to look at how you feel both mentally and physically is the first step in helping yourself to cope with stress. Yet most of us are so busy that we do not take the time to stop and listen to our bodies, and to ask ourselves, 'How do I feel right now?' We either ignore the niggling aches and pains and feelings of discomfort, or accept them as an inevitable part of life. Take a moment to ask yourself the following questions.

Do you ever suffer from any of the following **physical symptoms** at work?

- eye fatigue or strain
- headaches
- neck pain or stiffness
- shoulder tension
- wrist or finger pain
- lower or upper backache
- aching legs
- sore feet
- stiff joints, for example, knees and elbows
- cramped muscles
- nervous stomach, indigestion
- tiredness, bouts of yawning

Do you ever experience any of the following **feelings** at work?

- lethargy
- restlessness
- depression, negative feelings
- panic
- helplessness, inadequacy
- irritability
- boredom
- frustration, anger

And finally, do you ever:

- leave work feeling irritable and grumpy?
- take the frustrations of the day home with you?
- feel so tired when you get home you just collapse in a chair?

How many did you tick? However many, do not despair; none of the symptoms and feelings listed is inevitable. You can do something about them and you have already started – by reading this book!

THE 1990S WORK ENVIRONMENT

Let's take a look at the general work environment that prevails today. The pace of change, new technology, increasing competition in the marketplace and the effects of recession will all have an impact on your particular work situation. More often than not this will manifest itself upon you, the individual, as stress.

Modern technology has resulted in many jobs being redefined. In industry many traditionally manual tasks are now automated. Many manufacturing companies operate production lines to maximize efficiency and productivity. But this means that the worker performs just one small task before passing the product on to the next person in the line. Both these developments expose the worker to repetitive tasks in a static position.

In the office environment, the developments in communications technology – the availability of the facsimile machine, electronic mail and the mobile phone, and the latest computer technology, such as lap-top computers and phone-linked computer modems – have had a considerable impact. On one hand, it has removed the necessity for workers to be office-bound and has introduced the concept of the 'Virtual Office', where work can be carried out wherever you happen to be: at home, in a hotel room, or even when travelling. On the other hand, communications technology has reduced the need for face-to-face meetings, and to some extent has made jobs more office-bound.

Internationally, organizations have adopted new management trends including performance measurement, performance-related pay and continual improvement policies in their fight to survive in an increasingly competitive global market. Such trends put managers and workers under great pressure to meet targets and deadlines, often with fewer resources and in less time than before. In addition, the recent recession experienced by most countries has jeopardized job security.

It is not only workers in industry and commerce who are faced with stressful environments. Those in the public sector, such as teachers, and in some countries, nurses and doctors, also face new pressures. There is an international trend towards reduced public expenditure and in many countries, for example, the United Kingdom, Australia and New Zealand, a move towards privatization of public sector organizations. Coping with this pace of change, and often having to work with reduced resources, provides a stressful work environment for people within these professions.

The culture of work

Today's society is on the whole 'materialistic' and consumer-oriented. Success is often measured by what you own: property, cars, household gadgets, fashionable clothes and accessories. Many people put themselves under great pressure to work very hard to fund their desired lifestyle. Achievement at work also has a high status in today's society. Once someone at a party has asked what your name is, the next question is often: 'What do you do?' For many people, their work is not just the means to earn a living, but something that provides them with a status, an identity, and is as important to them as their family life. Such people put themselves under great pressure to achieve at work and demand a high degree of job satisfaction.

If you work only to earn money, have little job satisfaction and would rather not be working at all, this also is a source of stress. You may feel resentful or angry that you have to do something you do not want to do, and may spend the whole day watching the clock until it is time to go home.

Work environments must have some form of structure and discipline to achieve efficiency and productivity, but the level will vary between professions. Working within a structured framework can be a cause of stress, especially for those people who resent being controlled, monitored and told when to have a tea break. Many people do not like working for other people and find it hard to take orders and instructions, but unless you are self-employed this is the reality of the workplace. Again, for certain people this is a great cause of stress. Obviously it is important to try to choose a career that suits your temperament and you will find rewarding. Sadly this does not always happen, and many people are working in jobs in which, for whatever reason, they are unhappy.

Work environments will vary in the degree of formality, but usually workers have to conform to a certain code of conduct and behaviour. If something goes wrong or upsets you, you cannot have a tantrum, burst into tears or do whatever you might do if you were at home to release the tension. You must suppress your feelings and try to keep on working. This can be a major cause of stress, especially if you do not regularly de-stress yourself to get rid of these bottled-up emotions and tensions. In your life outside work, you probably give much care to creating a home environment that you find comfortable, and in choosing people you like to be with as friends and acquaintances. Unfortunately, we do have not such control at work. We will all at some stage have to operate within conditions with which we feel uncomfortable, and with people whom in normal circumstances we would rather avoid! Again, this situation is a potential cause of stress, especially if you are powerless to change it.

The underlying message of this book, however, is that even if you cannot change the situation, you can change your attitude towards it.

3

Physical Stress at Work

THE PHYSICAL NATURE OF WORK

Those aches and pains you often experience occur because of the physical nature of your work. Each job will have its own set of physical characteristics, and it would be impossible to consider all the variations that may exist within even just one profession. For simplicity, we will therefore categorize the different types of work according to four common physical characteristics. Many jobs will not fall under just one of these, but can have components of all of them.

Sitting or remaining static for long periods

Why is it a problem?
We do not usually think of sitting as a potentially dangerous activity! It is normally associated with relaxation; you have a 'sit down' to relax and rest your legs and feet. But, as the old adage goes, everything should be done in moderation – even sitting! Sitting for long periods is the problem, and is a major cause of physical problems in desk-bound and other seated work. Your body is designed to move; your whole skeletal and muscular structure is designed for this purpose. The body

thrives on movement and does not like remaining static in any position for long periods.

Examples of jobs
Desk-bound work: secretaries, accountants, computer operators, writers
Driving: travelling sales representatives, taxi, bus and train drivers, delivery work
Machine operators: sewing machinists, cash-till operators
Any other job involving a static position for a long time, for example, kneeling

Common problems
- **Long-term postural problems** Continual bad posture while sitting at work can result in your body assuming long-term postural problems, such as a stooped back or rounded shoulders. You increase the risk of this happening when no remedial action is taken, for example, if you do not exercise your body.
- **Neck pain and upper or lower backache** A common cause of such problems is bad posture while sitting and working at a desk or work station; for example, sitting hunched over your desk or twisting your neck to look at your computer screen.
- **Tense, cramped muscles** The muscles support and move the joints. When your body is immobile for long periods, you are not exercising your muscles. They are being held in a static position. As a result they can spasm and knot, causing that familiar muscle tension, cramp and aching.
- **Stiff joints** It is common for people who sit or kneel for long periods to suffer from stiff knees, elbows and ankles when they stand up and move around. This simply occurs due to lack of use.
- **Poor circulation** Movement aids circulation. When you move your body, the blood flow increases. It is obvious, therefore, that when you sit for a long time your circulation becomes more sluggish. At work, the position in which you

sit means your body is at right angles, often with your legs crossed. This restricts the flow of blood through the body and in particular to the lower limbs. This can result in numbness, particularly in your buttocks, and in cramp and pins and needles in your legs.

- **Feelings of lethargy and/or restlessness** Lethargy is a common side-effect of an inert body. Do you ever feel tired and lethargic at work even after a good night's sleep? This could be because the restricted blood flow has resulted in less oxygen being fed to the various parts of your body. As a result a general feeling of fatigue can flood the body. The breathing and the metabolic rate also slow, leaving you feeling drained of energy. Does this sound familiar? Sometimes you may experience an opposite reaction and feel restless and fidgety, irritable and unable to concentrate. This is usually experienced by people who have a naturally high level of energy that is being suppressed by sitting still.

Standing for long periods

Why is it a problem?
Many jobs will require long periods of standing. Common examples are shop staff, waiting staff and factory staff. The body is designed to move, and standing all day can cause as many problems as sitting or being in some other static position.

Examples of jobs
Shop work: sales assistants, floor managers
Catering: kitchen workers, waiting staff
Nursing
Hairdressers
Traffic wardens, police, security guards
Factory workers where work involves standing at a work station

Common problems
- **Postural problems** As the body tires from long periods of standing, good posture often suffers. The muscles of the back and stomach become tired from holding the body in alignment and the most common tendency is to arch the back, push the stomach forward and round the shoulders. This misalignment of the back commonly causes lower and middle backache. This can result in long-term postural problems. Poor posture when standing is exacerbated by wearing high heels.
- **Backache** Lower and middle backache is a common side-effect of long periods of standing, mainly due to poor posture. The backache may be caused at work, but will not automatically go away when you leave work and have a chance to relax and sit down.
- **Aching, sore legs and varicose veins** Standing for a long time puts enormous pressure on the legs. They have to bear the whole body's weight. Aching legs, swollen ankles and occasionally varicose veins are all common symptoms of standing for long periods.
- **Sore feet** As with the legs, standing for long periods puts the feet on the spot as they have to support the body's weight. As the body becomes more tired, so the weight is less supported and bears down on the feet. The result can be burning, aching and swollen feet. The choice of footwear can greatly affect this problem; ill-fitting shoes can cramp the feet, reducing the blood supply, and can also cause blisters, bunions, corns and other problems. High heels make the problem worse as the body's weight is centred on the ball of the foot.

Repetitive work

Why is it a problem?
Small repetitive tasks expose the worker to the risk of strain and injury. The body thrives on a variety of tasks and a repetitive

task such as keyboard work can overextend certain muscles and tendons in isolation, and can result in strain and injury.

Examples of jobs
Key board operators: secretaries, accountants, computer operators
Machine operators: till operators
Switchboard operators
Musicians
Sports professionals: golfers, snooker players
Any other repetitive task: writing, stuffing envelopes, stamping forms

Common problems
- **Repetitive Stress Injury (RSI)** RSI is now a common term. It embraces a number of local injuries, usually to the arms, wrists and fingers, ranging from temporary fatigue to peritendinitis and carpal tunnel syndrome. The main cause of such injuries is overuse of the muscles, tendons and ligaments coupled with being in a static position; for example, holding the body and arms stationary while performing limited movements with the fingers on a keyboard. Keyboard users are not the only sufferers of RSI; it can be caused by any similar repetitive task, such as repeated use of a foot pedal, or continually picking up the telephone receiver. It can also be caused by non-office activities, such as racket sports, playing musical instruments and even knitting!
- **Strain and injury** Repetitive movements work on particular muscle groups and joints and by simple overuse can result in strain and injury, such as tennis elbow, the term used to refer to injuries of the elbow joint due to repetitive movements such as experienced when playing tennis. Many jobs will expose the worker to repetitive movements: continually reaching up for something on a top shelf or bending to pick something off the floor; twisting your head to look in the

driver's mirror of your car; or hole-punching large quantities of papers.

Physically strenuous work

Why is it a problem?
If you exercise you will know that strenuous movements such as jogging, aerobics, playing sport and using weights can often result in stiffness or sore muscles, and can also carry a risk of injury. But you will also know how to protect yourself from injury by warming-up the muscles before exercise, by stretching afterwards and by not overextending yourself, but listening to your body to know when to stop. Some jobs involve physical work, but less attention is paid to safeguarding the body; you will probably not warm-up the muscles or stretch out at regular intervals and you may not be able to stop, but just have to keep going.

Examples of jobs
Lifting work: porters, delivery/removal workers, builders
Manual work: builders, car mechanics, gardeners, physiotherapists
Dancers
Sports professionals

Common problems
- **Muscle stiffness, strain and injury** Ranging from muscle fatigue and stiffness to pulled muscles and more serious injuries.
- **Joint problems** Knee problems, such as cartilage trouble, and wrist and elbow problems, such as tennis elbow.
- **Back problems** Commonly caused by incorrect lifting technique, and one major cause of absenteeism from work in the United Kingdom.

THE PHYSICAL WORK ENVIRONMENT

Your physical work environment – your equipment and its position, the lighting, ventilation and temperature – can affect your health and well-being. Sick Building Syndrome (SBS) has been recognized by the World Health Organization since 1982. Symptoms of SBS can include tiredness and lethargy, headaches, breathing problems and cold symptoms. Causes of SBS can include poor ventilation, temperature control and lighting and also problems caused by electromagnetic fields (EMFs), static electricity and fumes given from new paint, carpets and cleaning products. Every physical work environment will vary, but here are some common areas that can cause problems.

Working with display screen equipment (DSE)

Most office workers will encounter work with DSE. It may only be part of your job, or your whole day may revolve around DSE work. Looking at DSE for a long period can cause the following problems:

Common problems
- **Eye strain** You may feel a burning sensation in your eyes, particularly common among wearers of contact lenses, or your eye muscles may twitch. These are signs that your eyes are irritated or tired.
- **Headaches** Headaches can occur for a variety of reasons, but they can be a secondary symptom of eye strain. Working with a DSE may be a particular problem for migraine sufferers or for those who also work in badly lit offices. Nausea can also accompany headaches caused by too much DSE work.

Air conditioning/poor ventilation

Your work environment may have less than satisfactory ventilation. Basement offices and workplaces can have insufficient air circulation. Windows can open on to roads letting polluted air flood in; the atmosphere may be dusty due to lack of cleaning, or you may be exposed to passive smoking. Air conditioning is now common in many workplaces, but while it keeps the room at a regulated temperature it too may cause problems.

Common problems
- **Dehydration** Caused by too little moisture in the air because of air conditioning and can dry mucous membranes, eyes and skin.
- **Upper respiratory tract problems** Sore throats, tickling throats, breathing problems. Asthma or other breathing problems can be aggravated by poor ventilation or some air-conditioning systems.
- **Tiredness and excessive yawning** When you yawn, it is a signal that your body is striving for more oxygen to enter the bloodstream.

If you are exposed at work to any chemical or other type of fumes, for example, in a workshop or factory or in a smoking environment, it is particularly important that you have adequate ventilation.

Lighting

Natural light is the best light in which to work, but this is not always available. Many workplaces rely on artificial lighting to supplement the natural light or even to replace it. If lighting is not sufficient for the task, it can cause many problems.

Common problems
- **Headaches** Can be caused or aggravated by fluorescent or other types of lighting.

- **Eye problems** Eye strain, sore red eyes or twitching eye muscles can be a problem, if poor lighting is causing you to strain your eyes to focus on your work, be it a computer screen, manuscript or other task. Bright sunlight can also be a problem if it reflects off your DSE screen or work station and causes you to squint.

Noise

Nearly all jobs will expose the worker to some level of noise. This may be the noise of telephones and colleagues' voices; external noise such as traffic; or the noise of equipment and machinery. Noise levels become a problem if they affect your ability to work properly, for example, if they distract you from your task, make it impossible for you to be heard, or cause you to have physical side-effects. Workers in certain jobs will need to wear ear protection.

Common problems
- **Lack of concentration** If background noise is distracting you from your work.
- **Headaches** A headache is a typical body response to intrusive noise.
- **Hearing problems** Impaired hearing from high levels of noise, for example, from heavy machinery, is a very serious problem and can be permanent.

Health and safety

Different work environments will have particular health and safety requirements, for example, for jobs that involve working with potentially dangerous chemicals and equipment. The particular risk created by such work will be addressed by health and safety legislation in safety procedures and other requirements, such as training, supervision and protective clothing.

4

Mental Stress at Work

The causes and symptoms of mental stress are not as clear-cut as those for physical stress. They can creep up on you, and the effect can be cumulative. Mental stress can manifest itself in both physical and mental symptoms; for example, being under great pressure at work can make you feel anxious and irritable, but can also give you a headache, nervous stomach and tense shoulders. The causes can be many and the symptoms can be various. Sometimes you may not realize that mental stress was the cause of a particular physical problem. Whether you find a particular situation stressful, and how you react if you do, is important; everyone has a different stress tolerance level that will depend on many factors, including general health and personal happiness.

COMMON SYMPTOMS OF MENTAL STRESS

Symptoms of mental stress can be a range of negative feelings from anger to depression, or a whole set of physical problems from headaches to sleeping problems. Common symptoms of short-term stress are varied but may include:

- tense shoulders, neck and back
- headaches

- nervous stomach
- irritability
- depression
- feelings of helplessness
- lack of concentration
- feeling emotional and tearful

In the long-term, continual stress can result in, among others:

- general susceptibility to illness, ie repeated colds
- insomnia
- irritable bowel syndrome
- fertility problems
- cardiovascular problems, such as high blood pressure

CAUSES OF MENTAL STRESS AT WORK

So what is it at work that can make us vulnerable to the above symptoms? Every person will react differently to being under stress at work, and will find different situations stressful. However, we list here some common causes.

- **Working to deadlines and targets** Some people thrive on such pressure, but for many it creates a stressful situation. This is a particular problem when the deadlines or targets are not realistic and can lead to a range of feelings from helplessness, resentment and frustration to sheer panic.
- **Heavy workloads** Too much work and too little time in which to do it can result in panic and anxiety as well as feeling resentful and exploited.
- **Conflicts with colleagues** If you get on well with everyone at work, you are very lucky! Problematic work relationships are a common cause of stress. Personality clashes or differences of opinions with your work colleagues, your boss or your subordinates can greatly affect your health.
- **Dealing with difficult people** You may only deal occasionally with a difficult client or supplier, or it may be a central

part of your work if you work in such areas as services or personnel, or in a contentious occupation such as law or the tax office. Dealing with people who are rude, persistent or just plain awkward can be very stressful and upsetting. It is our natural reaction to take the offence personally, rather than in the capacity of our work, especially if we have not been given training or guidance on how to handle such situations.

- **Responsibility** Many jobs carry a degree of responsibility; responsibility for a budget, for a particular project, for a department or for other people. Many people enjoy responsibility, but it can also put you under pressure, especially if the responsibility is unwanted or if you are not sufficiently trained or experienced to handle it. This stress can be increased if an element of risk is involved, such as when you have to make a decision or agree a course of action, the results of which are not certain.

- **Job insecurity** This is a great cause of low morale and stress for many people, particularly during periods of economic recession. 'Jobs for life' is a thing of the past, and job security can no longer be taken for granted. Many people have to work with the knowledge that redundancies are a possibility within their organization.

- **Presentations and interviews** It is a normal reaction to become nervous and anxious before having to make a presentation, deliver a speech or attend an interview. A certain amount of nerves are necessary to get the adrenaline flowing and make you perform well. Symptoms of such apprehension may be a headache, upset stomach or irritability, and increased heart beat and breathing rate and actual shaking of the hands nearer the time of performance. Some people only get very nervous the first time they have to make a speech, but others will react this way every time no matter how they try to control it. If your job involves much of this type of work and you are frequently suffering from nerves it will contribute to a high stress level.

- **Distractions, poor organization and noise** We are all

greatly affected by our environment; by what other people are doing around us, by noise and by visual distractions. We need to concentrate when we work and a noisy work environment or one where other people are continually interrupting is a sure recipe for stress.

- **Lack of training** If you are expected to work in a job without being given sufficient training on, for example, equipment, machinery or work procedures, this can create a very stressful work environment. This may result in feelings of inadequacy, helplessness, panic or frustration.
- **Change** It is quite natural for many people to find change very stressful. Change at work may vary from a new job or work location to a new boss, new equipment, or just a different way of doing a particular task. Some people find change stimulating, but it is also common to feel unsettled, insecure and even threatened by change in the workplace.
- **Things going wrong** No matter how well organized you are there is always a chance that things can still go wrong! Not everything is within your control and dealing with unexpected crises is a major cause of stress.

WHY IS MENTAL STRESS A PROBLEM?

Stress caused by these work situations and by many others can translate into a number of physical symptoms. But how does this happen? When you are placed in a stressful situation, the mind sends messages to the body. There is a rapid increase in your metabolism and hormonal, physiological and biochemical changes take place in your body. Scientists call this the 'fight-or-flight' reaction. The body prepares to react; you will feel your heartbeat and breathing rate quicken and your muscles tense in preparation for activity as the blood is diverted to the major organs, the heart, lungs and muscles.

This is an appropriate reaction if you are going to engage in physical activity, either to fight or to run away. If this happened you would expend energy and then the body would return to normality. But usually there is no such activity. Your computer jams, you have a stressful telephone call, or you make a mistake and you do not leap into action; you will probably stay sitting down and continue working. The tension builds up and there is no release, no return to normality. You stay wound-up, and when you next encounter a stressful situation, the effect becomes cumulative. This is what makes stress so dangerous and why it is essential to de-stress yourself regularly.

You might not be able to change many of the factors that cause you problems in the office, but with a little effort you *can* change your attitude to work and the way in which you cope with stressful situations.

5

How Yoga Can Help

Hatha yoga is a holistic system of exercise. It works on the body and on the mind. We have seen in the previous chapters how your physical work environment can cause problems such as back pain, eye strain or repetitive strain injuries. We have also seen how the mental stress caused by work can result in physical and mental symptoms.

The body and mind are totally interdependent. When you are under pressure, your mind sends messages to your body saying 'I'm stressed out – help!', and the body reacts. Similarly, feelings of physical discomfort and pain can affect how you feel mentally. The body and mind have to work in harmony and that is why yoga is the perfect solution for workplace stress. The basis of hatha yoga is union of the mind and body. A healthy body results in well-being of the mind and vice versa.

Let us take a closer look at how yoga can actually help you tackle the unwanted side-effects of your work. The yoga exercises can help in several ways:

- the physical exercises can generally relieve body tension, ease stiffness and increase your energy and also help specific problems, such as backache and eye strain
- the relaxation, breathing and meditation exercises can help you tackle the effects of mental stress
- regular practice of the physical, breathing, relaxation and

meditation exercises can help you to be more resistant to the side-effects of workplace stress and better able to cope with the problems it poses

- regular practice of the exercises will induce a sense of general well-being that will affect your whole life
- yoga will teach you how to observe how you feel and be more in tune with your body and its needs

The exercises in this book have been especially selected and adapted to help people at work. There are many areas in which yoga can help you and we outline the main benefits below:

- **Relief from stiff joints and muscles** If you are sitting or in any static position for a long time you will experience a general stiffness of the joints. The yoga exercises will gently limber up your body, easing the joints back into action and will increase your general mobility and suppleness. Yoga works on a system of balance; if you stretch one way, you must counteract the stretch the other way. For example, if you sit hunched over your work station with your back rounded for a long time, a gentle yoga stretch backwards will release the stiffness and tension that will have accumulated.

  The yoga exercises will also stretch out muscles that have been cramped in one position. Tense muscles restrict the flow of blood. As they stretch, there will be a release of tension and the blood flow will increase through your body.

  A supple spine is essential to good health. Many of the exercises concentrate on improving the flexibility and condition of the spinal column and surrounding muscle groups.

- **Help with postural problems** Yoga demands good posture. The starting point for every exercise is for the back, neck and head to be in a straight line, with the stomach muscles held firm. You will see later that every exercise starts with this posture check. By carrying out the exercises regularly, you will re-educate your body to hold itself straight whilst at work and so prevent the aches and pains associated with recurrent poor posture. The exercises will also make you more aware of your body and of whether you are sitting or standing correctly, so you can check your posture throughout the day.

- **Increase your circulation** We have mentioned how by stretching the muscles and releasing tension, the flow of blood around the body is increased. In addition, remaining in any static position, especially sitting, restricts the circulation. All the exercises in this book require you to move your body and for one section we ask you to stand up and give the body a good stretch. As a result, the exercises will increase your circulation and boost your energy levels.

- **Reduce the risk of RSI** If practised regularly, the wrist, finger and arm exercises included in this book will reduce the risk of RSI. They mobilize the joints, stretch the tendons that have been locked in one position and increase the circulation to the area at risk.

- **Ease eye strain** You may be surprised to find out that yoga includes exercises for the eyes. Other forms of exercise usually ignore the eyes. Have you ever thought to exercise yours? Yet the eyes are essential organs with many muscles that, like others in the body, tire from overuse. The eye exercises in this book release the tension and strain that can accumulate from long periods staring at a computer screen, peering at text or other close-up work and coping with poor lighting conditions.

- **Revitalize the body** When you do yoga exercises, you release tension. This will free vast resources of energy, energy that your stress was consuming. When you do the physical exercises, you will also increase the blood flow to the body. The blood carries oxygen and nourishes the cells. The breathing exercises will charge the body with increased oxygen, dispel toxins that have accumulated in the body and leave you feeling full of energy again.

- **Release of physical tension caused by stress** Your upper back, neck and shoulders will be the first place where tension gathers. The result can be knotted and aching muscles that will feel tender to touch. Many of the exercises included in the book concentrate on this area, loosening knotted muscles and dispersing tension – like giving yourself a massage.

- **Alleviate feelings of stress** The focus on breathing throughout all the exercises, and the specific breathing exercises, will calm you. Regulated breathing has a powerful effect on the body. It calms the nerves and stabilizes the emotions. In addition the increased oxygen supply will make you feel more alert.

  The relaxation and meditation exercises will focus your mind and enable the whole body to relax, dispelling the tension that has mounted during the day, leaving you feeling serene and in control.

- **General feeling of well-being** This will be the cumulative effect of regular yoga practice.

6

How to Improve Your Workplace

No two workplaces will be exactly the same. But here we look at the basic components of your workplace and consider how you can make small changes to improve your well-being at work.

You might have heard of the word 'ergonomics', which is the relationship between you and your workplace. Ergonomics in practice is for you and your employers to look at the design of work equipment and systems so that they combine efficiency and reduce the risk of stress and injury.

In most countries, employers are bound by law to provide a safe environment for you to work in. If any part of your work, or any area of your equipment, is causing you stress or pain you should tell your supervisor, personnel manager, or employer immediately and ask that the problem is addressed. This might be something as simple as a new chair, or it might require the re-design of a work system or procedure, for example, for a team of workers to alternate between computer work and telephone work to reduce the risk of eye strain and repetitive stress injury. Even the smallest physical discomfort – a wobbly table surface or a chair seat that is too high or low – can greatly affect your comfort, your concentration and as a result your performance. It is therefore in your employer's best interests to provide you with a safe and comfortable work environment.

EQUIPMENT

Every workplace and every job will require particular equipment ranging from the desktop computer to complex factory machinery to pen and paper or a hairdryer. We could not possibly begin to look at all these variations, but here we concentrate on core equipment which will be common to many types of job.

Your chair

Many jobs are predominantly sedentary. It makes sense then, that your chair is a vital piece of equipment. If it is uncomfortable or faulty, there is a risk of postural problems. Different jobs will require different types of seating facilities; the ideal chair for keyboard work will be different from that for working on a production line or sitting at a cash till in a shop. As every job will be different, so is every person. People are different heights and have different length legs, and your chair should be able to adapt to accommodate these variations. As a general guideline, your chair should have the following facilities:

- adjustment for seat height
- adjustment for angle and height of back rest
- good lumbar support
- adequate cushioning in the seat and back to absorb shock

Depending on your job, your chair may also need to be able to swivel from side to side and have wheels for mobility.

The seat depth should be sufficient to support your legs from the hip to the knee. There should be no pressure at the back of the knee or middle of the thigh. Some chairs may have arm rests, but these are not necessary. The seat of the chair should be able to tilt forward slightly so the pelvis can tilt. Some chairs have a semi-automatic rocking facility. The ideal chair for desk work would have five castors to allow free movement.

Your chair should enable you to sit for considerable lengths of time in comfort. If you are experiencing any discomfort or pain ask for your chair to be looked at and if necessary request a replacement. Remember that your spine is the nerve centre of the body; it is essential that it is supported and cushioned by your chair.

Your desk

Your desk should be large enough for your computer keyboard, telephone and any other equipment, and leave you adequate room for documents to be freely positioned. Your computer should be placed so that the cables are not dangling where they may be knocked or tripped over, but are secured. If you are typing from or referring to source documents frequently, you should ask for a document holder. This holds the documents vertical and means you do not have to keep looking down, a movement which can put pressure on the neck and upper back. There should be adequate leg room under your desk to enable you to take up a variety of leg positions.

Your Display Screen Equipment (DSE)

DSE is used in a range of jobs: for word processing, for computerized accounts, for computer design, for desktop publishing, stock records and a multitude of other tasks. If you use a DSE, it should have the following facilities:

- adjustment for contrast and brightness
- the keyboard and screen should be able to be moved independently
- angle adjustment for the screen so it can be tilted or swivelled as necessary
- flaps for the keyboard so it can be tilted

- there should be enough room in front of your keyboard to enable you to have support for your hands and arms when necessary

It is important that there is no glare or reflection off your screen as this can cause eye strain. Turn off your screen and check it for glare. If you can see your reflection, you need to reposition it or change the source of light; your machine should be at right-angles to any natural light in order to minimize any glare. You should not work at DSE which is directly in front of, or opposite a window. Make sure the windows have blinds so you can cut out sunlight if necessary.

Light can also reflect off any shiny smooth surface such as filing cabinets, desk tops or glass partitions, and affect your screen viewing.

Artificial lighting can also cause reflections off the screen. Experiment with your lighting. Uplighters or similar diffuse the light and result in less glare than traditional fluorescent lighting.

If you are unable to minimize the glare, you could ask for an anti-glare screen. But this should really be a last resort as you are only limiting the side-effects of the existing problem.

If there is any flickering of your screen image, call a technician immediately as working with this can strain your eyes. Remember to clean your screen regularly. Computer screens attract dust and grime easily and this can impair your view of the screen.

Take care over the choice of colours on your screen. Bright fluorescent colours may be fun but over time can strain your eyes.

Many employers offer free eye tests for employees who use DSE as a substantial part of their job (in some countries, such as the United Kingdom, it is obligatory by law). If you require glasses for the purpose of DSE work only, your employers may contribute towards the cost. If you experience any eye strain, visual problems or headaches it is important that you have an eye test.

POSTURE AT WORK

Sitting

Correct posture can help prevent the muscular-skeletal problems that sedentary work can cause. The following is a posture guide for sitting at your desk and undertaking keyboard work, but many of the points are also relevant for any desk work:

- Adjust your seat height, so that when you are seated your forearms are horizontal and the wrists are straight when using your keyboard.
- Your feet should be flat on the floor. If they are not, you should use a footrest. If a footrest is used when it is not needed, this can cause postural problems.
- Do not twist or cross your legs. This can twist the pelvis and restrict circulation.
- Do not perch on the end of your seat. Sit back so the chair back provides support for your lumbar region.
- If it is more comfortable, you could put a cushion in the small of your back.
- When you use your keyboard, there should be minimal extension, flexion and deviation of the wrists.
- Avoid sitting in the same position for a long period of time; break for 10–30 seconds every ½ hour. Stretch and relax.

Standing

When we have to stand for long periods of time, the body becomes fatigued and good posture suffers. It is most common for people to arch their lower back and relax the stomach muscles, putting extra weight on the pelvis and hip area and to stoop and round their shoulders and neck. Standing for long periods also puts great pressure on the feet which are bearing the whole weight of the body. It is common for the balls of the feet or the heels to feel sore and burn. Sometimes to relieve the discomfort we put weight on other parts of the foot, for example the outside, and this in turn can affect our posture.

- Try to be aware of your posture and do regular posture checks. Just to remind yourself – shoulders back; stomach in – at intervals during the day will make a difference and help you to re-educate your muscles into holding good posture.
- Movement helps greatly. If possible, walk around regularly or, if not, shift the weight from one foot to the other, clench and release your toes within your shoes and, if footwear permits, raise the body up onto the tips of the toes.
- Footwear: the choice of footwear is vitally important for jobs that involve standing for long periods. High heels for women are not a good idea; the whole weight of the body is centred on the ball of the foot and they also affect the alignment of the pelvis. Some women, however, may find flat-heeled shoes uncomfortable if they have a tight Achilles' tendon and will find a slight heel preferable. Shoes that support and cushion the foot will be best. Shoes that pinch or cramp the foot will cause unnecessary discomfort. Different jobs will have different dress codes or safety requirements that will affect choice of footwear. Some jobs involve a uniform, or you may have to wear a safety shoe.

TAKING BREAKS

You may not have any control over your work routine, but if you do, make the most of this freedom to maximize your well-being at work. The key is variety: variety of task will keep your mind alert and will prevent many of the physical problems associated with repetitive work. In many instances it is a case of just listening to your body. If your eyes are straining from reading a document or working on a computer screen take a break and do something different; make a few telephone calls or do some filing. If your legs feel cramped and your back aches, carry out a task or errand that involves standing up and walking. We realize that you may be under pressure to finish a particular task by a given deadline, but remember just a few minutes' break will result in you being fresher and able to work more effectively.

In particular, working for long periods on DSE can put you at risk of suffering from postural problems, eye strain and repetitive stress injury. You are also likely to suffer from general fatigue and lapses of concentration. It is important that you should take regular breaks from your DSE work. This might be to carry out other tasks or, if you have no other work to do, to move away from the screen for a rest period.

The timing of such breaks is very important. You should not break when you are already fatigued and suffering discomfort. This is too late. You should have short frequent breaks. Everyone's tolerance will be different and your employers should allow you the flexibility to take breaks at your discretion.

PHYSICAL CONDITIONS

Noise

Noise can be a stress factor in many workplaces. Office equipment, such as printers and photocopiers, will make some noise, but this should not be so intrusive that it impairs your concentration or requires you to raise your voice to be heard on the telephone or by colleagues. In industrial workplaces, machinery may be very noisy and can impair concentration and result in headaches. In many cases where it is not possible to reduce the noise levels, ear protection may be a requirement of the job. Here are some basic tips to help reduce the noise levels in your workplace, particularly in the office environment:

- try repositioning noisy equipment so it is as far away from your work station as possible
- use an acoustic shield for your printer; these are available for most models

- install a partition screen around the photocopier or printer or other noisy equipment
- reduce the level of your phone's ringing tone
- ask for double glazing to reduce external noise
- ask for air conditioning so that windows do not have to be opened letting in road and other external noise

Lighting

Poor lighting in any workplace can result in eye strain and headaches if it is not adequate for you to carry out your work. Lighting should be appropriate for the task; for example, darker ambient light for computer work and brighter light for paperwork or other close work. Fluorescent lights produce a harsh light; if you are stuck with them try taking out one of the tubes to lessen the glare. Consider as an alternative using uplighters that diffuse the light, or task lighting, ie desk lamps. Try to avoid fluorescent and halogen lights for desk lights as they emit a large amount of electromagnetic fields (EMFs). EMFs are thought to be capable of causing headaches and other health-related problems.

Remember that white is reflective and white walls, filing cabinets and even white paper will reflect light. Similarly, glass panelling will reflect light around the room.

Temperature/humidity

The temperature of the workplace should be comfortable for its workers. As a general guide, it should be between 66–73°F. If you have air conditioning, a thermostat will monitor the temperature. If you do not, it will be a matter of controlling the heating and opening windows to maintain a comfortable temperature. If overheating is a problem in the summer months, portable fans and air-conditioning units can be hired.

If there is a lack of fresh air in your office, make sure you go out for a walk in your lunch period.

If the air is too dry, you might suffer a tickly throat, dry eyes and skin. This is a side effect of some air-conditioning systems. Indoor plants help to restore humidity, as does a bowl of water placed in the office. You can also buy humidifiers.

HEALTH AND SAFETY LEGISLATION

Most countries have health and safety at work legislation which provides guidelines for these areas and also sets minimum requirements. Many employers will make this information available to their employees and will have representatives who come and check your work station and make sure that the guidelines are implemented and maintained. If, however, your employer is less willing to address problems to do with your work environment, this information is usually readily available and you can use it to strengthen your request for improvements. It is very short-sighted of any employer to overlook staff well-being at work. Workers who have a comfortable and safe work environment will be far more productive and less likely to leave than those who do not. In the long term it is therefore financially beneficial for employers to invest in their employees' welfare at work.

7

What to Eat at Work

'You are what you eat' is a common adage, but how much thought do you give to what you eat and drink at work? What you eat and drink can greatly affect your performance at work. In the short term, your diet can affect your energy levels, your efficiency and even your moods. In the long term, an imbalanced diet can have serious health consequences.

It is easy to get into bad eating habits at work. Many people will find it tempting to snack throughout the day. This could be because you are bored, or to comfort yourself if you are feeling under stress, or you may find you occasionally crave something sweet to boost your energy levels. This is particularly easy if there is a canteen, tea trolley or shop nearby. Many people are so busy that they do not find the time for a lunch break and miss this meal altogether, or just snack on junk food.

There are many books that look specifically at nutrition and provide advice on what to eat and what not to eat. The purpose of this chapter is to make you pause for a moment to think about what you do eat and drink at work and see if there is any room for improvement, and to provide you with some simple tips and guidance.

- **Have a good breakfast** You are probably very familiar with this piece of advice, but the reality is that we often rush to work with only a cup of coffee or tea inside us. Breakfast is a vital meal; if you miss it you might not have eaten for over twelve hours by the time you get to work in the morning. You then expect your body and mind to perform well, which is like expecting a car to drive without fuel! Breakfast will give you a good start to the day, especially if there is a chance that you might be too busy to have a proper lunch, and it will help prevent the temptation to snack on sugary snacks between meals.

Breakfast should be a nutritious and balanced meal. For the hearty appetite this could be a full cooked breakfast but if you do choose this option make sure you grill rather than fry, and try to limit a cooked breakfast to once or twice a week. A more healthy option would be something simpler like orange juice and cereal or toast (preferably brown). Go for high-fibre cereals rather than those with added sugar. Have skimmed or semi-skimmed milk on your cereal and in tea, and choose a low-fat spread for your toast. An alternative choice for breakfast would be a selection of fresh fruit with low fat yoghurt. Hot water with a little lemon juice is an excellent drink for when you first wake up. It cleanses the body and aids the elimination of toxins.

To have breakfast, you might have to get up earlier in the morning, but do try and be disciplined. There is a danger that if you do miss breakfast, due to lack of time, you might become desperately hungry en route to work and resort to buying chocolate or something similar to keep you going until lunch. Try and be organized and have a supply of something a little more nutritious at work, such as cereal bars, rice cakes, fruit, bagels or yoghurt, so you can eat something when you arrive.

- **Drink throughout the day** When you feel thirsty, it actually means your body is already dehydrated. It is important to drink regularly throughout the day. Do not just drink coffee and tea but try to drink water as well. If possible, have a bottle on your desk or work station or in your car. Water cleanses the body and is the best thirst quencher. Try to avoid sweet drinks, like coke or lemonade. These, apart from being loaded with calories, pump up your blood sugar and do not really quench your thirst. If you are not keen on water, try a low-sugar fruit squash.

- **Try to quit the coffee** Coffee is sometimes referred to as the 'pick-me-up-drop-me-down' drink. Coffee contains caffeine, and caffeine is a drug. It gives you a short-lived boost by stimulating the nervous system. You temporarily feel that you are more clear-headed, alert and energetic, but in reality it impairs your mental performance. It stimulates your central nervous system, pancreas, heart and cerebral cortex. It makes the heart beat rapidly and irregularly and too much coffee over time could contribute to high blood pressure.

  Try to reduce your intake of coffee; drink decaffeinated, or switch to herbal or fruit teas. You may feel headachy, irritable or even shaky when you first quit, but this will only be temporary. Persevere – it will be worth it. Remember that tea too has substantial amounts of caffeine, if less than coffee, so avoid excessive tea drinking.

- **Beware of sugary snacks** Sugar, unless from natural foods such as fruit, has the potential to make you feel tired, depressed and emotionally unstable. This is because raised blood sugar triggers insulin imbalances within the body. Sugar may give you a temporary feeling of energy and well-being. Some people miss meals and snack on chocolate because it gives them energy. But, despite the claims made by some confectioners, chocolate is of little value nutritionally. After the blood sugar has been raised, it can plummet back down leaving you with headaches and mood swings. This is quite apart from the long-term health problems of excessive sugar intake, ie dental and weight problems.

  If you crave for sweet things during the day, try eating dried or fresh fruit. The sugar in fruit is fructose and is not a refined sugar. It will give you energy, but the body has to work harder to get this from the food, unlike the instant fix of refined sugar snacks. Wean yourself off chocolate slowly;

that way you are more likely to stick to your reformed eating habits.

- **Eat a balanced lunch** You may go out for lunch, visit the work canteen or gobble a sandwich at your desk or work station or in your car. Whatever you do, give a little thought to what you eat. A balance of starch, fibre and protein is the ideal lunch. Examples of a balanced lunch would be:

—wholemeal bread sandwich with salad and/or tuna, cottage cheese or low-fat cheese (Edam, feta, mozzarella), lean ham or chicken; avoid sandwich fillings with mayonnaise
—baked jacket potato with salad, tuna or baked beans
—mixed salad with pasta (leftovers can be used) and pitta bread
—baked beans on toast

If you eat in the canteen or go out to restaurants, beware of eating too heavy a meal. Always avoid rich creamy sauces and opt for low-fat sauces and have salad. Eating large and/or rich cooked meals can result in a feeling of sluggishness or abdominal discomfort as the metabolism slows down and your body attempts to digest the food as you sit at your desk or work station.

- **The urge to snack** It is an accepted fact that when we are bored we feel more hungry and eat more. Some people will also comfort eat when they are under stress. If you have an irresistible urge to snack between meals, try to avoid sugary and calorie-laden snacks. Snack on fresh or dried fruit. If you feel genuinely hungry between meals, eat something substantial like a sandwich or a bagel, crackers or rice cakes. This will be preferable to eating large amounts of foods of nutritionally low value, such as crisps or confectionery.

Some people, in particular women, may suffer from low blood sugar. This can mean that you will need to snack at regular intervals during the day to avoid becoming dizzy, shaky and irritable. If you do think you suffer from this, go to see your doctor who will advise you on how to cope.

Remember that imbalanced nutrition can be the cause of you feeling under par or having a low resistance to stress. Eat well and sensibly and you are better equipping your body to counter stress.

- **Make time to stop to eat** Many people do not take a set lunch break, but eat on the job. Although this is preferable to not eating at all, it can cause problems. If you gobble down your food whilst doing another task there is a danger that you are unlikely to chew your food and you will swallow it too quickly, both of which can cause indigestion. Try and stop even for just five or ten minutes to relax and eat your lunch.

- **Avoid alcohol** Some jobs might involve social drinking at lunchtime, or the business lunch when you may feel it would be impolite not to have one drink. Many jobs, particularly those that involve working with machinery, will have a ban on the consumption of alcohol during working hours. Drinking at lunch time is not a good idea, even if you just have to return to the office to work on the computer, or make a few telephone calls. Even the smallest amount of alcohol can make you feel drowsy and can impair your concentration and judgement. Alcohol also causes dehydration, so if you do have to indulge in a drink make sure you drink plenty of water afterwards.

- **Skipping meals** You may feel that skipping breakfast or lunch will cut down on your calorie intake and help weight control. This is not so! Long gaps between meals causes your body to slow down its rate of energy turnover (metabolism) and to switch to 'starvation mode'. The next time you eat, the body will immediately store it as fat: this is the body's way of looking after itself and conserving energy. Therefore, if you skip meals you are more likely to convert what you do eat into fat. It is far better to eat regularly, at least three (small) meals a day to keep your metabolism ticking over.

In general:

- stick to a low-fat, high-carbohydrate diet (pasta, rice, bread, potatoes)
- choose low fat options when available
- eat fresh fruit and salad
- drink plenty throughout the day, preferably water
- have breakfast and don't skip meals

8

The Yoga Approach to Work

You will probably spend around seven hours a day at work, which may be longer than the time you spend with your family and friends. We are used to thinking in terms of our personal life and putting effort and energy into making this happy and rewarding, but we tend to give little thought to our happiness at work. We think we have no control over the work situation and how it makes us feel and we just put up with it. It tends to be the norm to complain about work, and we often think that people who actually enjoy their occupation are in the minority and are lucky.

Work and how it makes you feel can greatly affect the rest of your life. If you are going home in the evenings and at weekends feeling under stress and irritable, worrying about work and dreading going back, it will affect your family and your friends. It will also influence the quality of your free time; if work is draining all your energy, you will have none left for the rest of your life. In this chapter we look at how you can make your time at work less stressful mentally. We realize that you might not be able to alter many of the things that cause you stress, but often simple changes of attitude and approach can make you cope with them better and feel more in control.

STRESS IN THE WORKPLACE

Different causes of stress

We can divide stress at work into two types. The external stress factors such as noise, equipment, workload and so on, and internal stress factors, such as our attitudes about ourselves and how we react to other people. This chapter will focus on the latter; on how we feel at work and how we can work towards feeling happier and more positive.

Your job will be one of the major influences on your life. Many of us are ambitious, and see our jobs as an important and fulfilling part of our life. For others, work is just a means to an end, somewhere you go to earn money so you can exist and enjoy your leisure hours and your time away from work. Neither of these approaches is right or wrong. What is important, though, is that we maintain a balance between work and rest, and between stress and relaxation. This balance may be different for each of us.

A certain amount of stress is necessary to perform well. It is natural to feel nervous before an important meeting, or when you are dealing with a crisis or problem. This stress is appropriate for the task and is not a problem as long as you do not remain in this state, but return to normal after the task has been completed. Stress becomes a problem when the pressure mounts beyond this healthy stimulus and the balance is lost. This could be, for example, because you react stressfully to an ongoing problem at work and there is no let-up. You might not even be able to identify these particular problems at first. You might not realize that your headaches, tension and moodiness are a reaction to this, and are symptoms of stress.

Self-observation

A starting point is self-observation. Observation and self-awareness are key points in yoga. Before you leave for work, sit and observe how you feel and mentally prepare yourself for the day ahead. Look at how you feel at work and how you react to things, and in this way you should be able to pinpoint your particular stressors. These will be unique to you. Everyone's tolerance levels will be different, and your own may even vary from day to day depending on other factors in your life, such as your health, your personal happiness and style of living.

Identify what creates stress for you

It would be impossible to address all the potential causes of workplace stress in this chapter, and a situation that one person finds stressful another might not. Some common reasons for stress at work may be quite fundamental, for example, you feel the job does not suit your temperament, or that you are overextended or bored. Your stress may stem from feelings of insecurity, or frustration because you do not have a clear career path or you are unsure about what expectations are being made of you. On the other hand, it could be something more specific; you may not get on with a particular colleague, you may be given unrealistic targets or deadlines, or you may not have been trained sufficiently on the new equipment in your office.

Other stress factors could be due to the nature of your work. You may have to deal with difficult customers, to meet strict deadlines or to sort out crises on a regular basis. Or you could be stressed because of competition among colleagues, office or work politics or harassment. Even the smallest things may affect you, for example, the way a colleague slurps his or her coffee or hums to him- or herself.

Sit and think for a while about what causes you stress. If it helps write a list of things that annoy and upset you. Try to be as specific as possible when you identify your stressor. For example, if it is your boss who causes you stress, try and think why and to identify the instances in which this happens.

What is your reaction to stress at work?

When you have identified your potential stressors, you have
already regained some control. You now have an idea of what
affects you. Look at how you react to these stress factors: does
your head ache, your pulse race, your jaw stiffen, your stomach
knot? If you have had a bad day at work, how do you feel
when you go home? Do you feel tired or hyperactive, irritable
or depressed? How do you sleep on those nights? Make a
mental note of these reactions.

Dealing with the stress

Think now whether you can do anything positive about your
personal stress factors. Remember that you are in control, and
try and think if you can take any action to improve the situation. Possible solutions could vary from the drastic action of
applying for a new job, to talking through a conflict with a
work colleague or to just asking for more training. If you
honestly feel you cannot do anything to improve the situation
then do not despair; you can still change how you react to it.

If you practise the yoga exercises included in this book regularly you will begin to feel differently. The combination of the
exercises will relax you, physically and mentally. When you are
relaxed you will react better to stress, interact better with your
colleagues, respond more positively to challenges and generally perform more efficiently. If you retain inner harmony and
peace, this will not only affect your own performance but also
the performance of those around you. You will find you
become more tolerant and more able to see people's good
points. It will also be easier to put work into perspective and to
remember that it is only a part of your life. That part will be as
important to you as you want it to be.

Uncertainty about the future is a major cause of stress. Will I
still have my job? Will I be promoted in the future? Or even
more short-term worries: Will the meeting go well tomorrow?

Will I meet this week's target? A solution to this is to live in the present. Yoga can help you do this; yoga philosophy concentrates on the present. There will, obviously, need to be a certain amount of planning ahead, but not an undue amount of projecting ourselves forward into often hypothetical situations. We will give 100 per cent to now, to the present. In yoga, people are encouraged to be responsible, dependable and honest, but not futuristic.

Emotion is not always easy to deal with, but it is important to vent your anger or grief and work through your feelings. If you do not do this, but hold onto your emotion, it often results in resentment and bitterness which then affects your attitudes to the people with whom you work and live.

How to minimize the stress – simple changes of attitude

- **Take criticism** Do not immediately react defensively. Evaluate the criticism and, whether you discard it or take it on board, see it as a positive action. There is positive criticism and painful criticism; identify which it is and then deal with it accordingly. Try not to take criticism of your work too personally. If someone complains that you work slowly, disagrees with a decision you have made or corrects something you have done, it does not mean you are a lesser person. See it in the context of your whole life and not just your job.
- **Have goals** Your job may provide goals for you in the form of targets or deadlines. These are very important, as long as they are realistic, as a form of motivation and for personal development. If your work does not provide them, make your own and monitor your progress.
- **Be open** Lack of communication is the downfall of many relationships, both professional and personal. You owe it to yourself to be open, to tell people how you feel, what you want to do. Your feelings are valid. If someone or something upsets you at work do not see it as a personal weakness.

Try to express yourself openly and honestly to minimize hostility and antagonism. Bottling up how you feel about even the smallest thing can lead to resentment and frustration, and the initial feeling can grow out of all proportion.

- **Clarify areas of disagreement** Do not let conflicts simmer away. Take control and try to openly identify the area of disagreement. This will be one positive step. You might even both agree on what you disagree about!

- **Live in the present – here and now** Do not dwell in the past. If you make a mistake, or feel you could have done something better than you did, just learn from it and move on. You need all your energy for the present. Let us live in the present. We can learn from past mistakes, but only through the present can we create a future. Do not fret about the future; it is natural for most of us to want to plan ahead, but do this positively. The future is by its very nature uncertain; worrying about it will not change this.

- **Work and act methodically** If your thoughts are unfocused and disordered, try and be outwardly methodical in your work. Write lists of things to do and prioritize these. Always try and finish one task before moving on to the next. Pause to consider your reaction before speaking or acting.

- **Consider the choices** When you are dealing with a certain situation, always systematically identify the problem and consider the choices of action. Remember you are in control and you will have a choice. The choice might not be to act at all, but this will still be a positive action.

- **Acknowledge your weaknesses** Be honest to yourself and acknowledge your weaknesses. If you come to terms with them and work within your limitations, you will be less vulnerable to criticism and less likely to disappoint yourself. Remember everyone has weaknesses; it does not devalue you or lessen your credibility.

- **Stay neutral and detached** If you are involved in a conflict situation it is very easy to become emotionally involved and react personally. It is easier said than done, but if you can remain neutral and try to assess the problem objectively it will be resolved much more easily and you will be far less stressed.

- **Have good time management** Many people become stressed because they seem to have too much to do and too little time. The full in-tray seen out of the corner of the eye can strike panic inside you, and if the phone keeps ringing and people keep giving you more work the situation can become too much. If you pause for a moment and plan your time, you will feel you have gained control. Prioritizing your work and deciding how much time you will spend on each task/activity will also help enormously. Rather than jumping from one task to another, work your way through the list systematically.

- **Prepare yourself for important tasks** If you have to make telephone calls which may be awkward or which will involve passing on or receiving information, take time to prepare yourself. Jot down notes of what you have to say and to ask for and try to anticipate responses. This will make you more relaxed and in control. The more prepared you are, the less likelihood there is of being caught unawares by unforeseen circumstances or things going wrong.

- **Do not be intimidated by your boss** It is important to have respect for your boss, as indeed for all your work colleagues, but to let yourself feel intimidated by them just because of their position is destructive. If you have a problem at work, the best solution is to discuss it with your boss. Even if it is not resolved, then at least he/she will be aware of the problem and can support you.

Some practical tips for creating a harmonious work environment

- **Visual stimulation** Consider how you can brighten up your workplace. Redecoration of your office will probably be a management decision, but if this is not practical perhaps you could go for simpler options and add some house plants or flowers, or put up some inspiring posters or quotes on your notice board. These are only cosmetic changes, but even a photograph of a loved one on your desk can make quite a difference.

- **Massage** Some organizations, particularly in the United States, have realized the benefits of massage and employ the services of on-site masseurs to relax their staff. This varies from giving head and neck massages to staff at their desk or work station, to being taken into a specially designated room for a longer session. Why not ask your employer to consider this?

- **Aromatherapy** Consider using an aromatherapy burner to fill your workplace with the pleasant scents of the many oils available. Pure aromatherapy oils have different effects; some are uplifting, others are relaxing and some have specific benefits such as disinfecting the air or helping to clear the sinuses. One thing aromatic oils all have in common is that they smell good! You can get special vaporizers that run off electricity or simple burners that use nightlights.

A final word – keep the stress in perspective

Finally, remember that you have control over your stress problem. You are bigger than the stress and the solution often lies within you. Try to think of the worst thing that can happen at work. It will probably be that you would be made redundant or sacked. Put this into perspective. Would it really be that bad? You would still be alive; you would still have your health, your family and friends. Try to think positively about how you would cope if this did happen. Once you have considered this worst possibility and realized that you could cope and you would survive the situation, it should make you feel in control. Your work is important, but remember it is only *part* of your life, not your *whole* life.

9

On-the-Spot Help for the Most Common Problems

This chapter deals with the most common problems that you may encounter during a busy working day. If you carry out the yoga work programmes regularly, you will find you will become less prone to the symptoms of stress at work. But there will still be times when you suffer from a particular problem and would welcome some instant relief. These yoga exercises can also be used individually for on-the-spot relief. We have taken eleven common physical and mental problems, indicated which of the yoga exercises will be particularly helpful for this complaint, and given you our top tip to help you tackle the problem on the spot at work.

When you have a headache or a backache at work, it is easy to reach for the painkillers. This will give you temporary relief from the discomfort and will mask the symptoms, but it will not get to the cause of the problem. So before you take something, give some thought to *what* might have caused the problem and try out the yoga options listed here. The relief might not be as instant, but in the long term it will be more natural and longer lasting.

The problem	Possible work-related causes	Yoga exercises to help	Quick fix
Headache	DSE work Poor lighting Poor ventilation Noise Mental stress; tension, anxiety, anger, frustation, panic Diet	Eye exercises Neck and head rotation Temple and head massage Calming breath Full breath Relaxation Meditation	With your eyes closed, massage your temples with your fingertips. As you do so breathe deeply in and out, making the outward breath twice as long as the inward breath, (say 3 counts in and 6 counts out).
Neck, shoulder and upper back tension	Poor posture Keyboard work Writing Driving Manual work Mental stress	Neck and head rotation Shoulder rotation Shoulder and arm rotation Chest expansion Forward bend with chest expansion (standing)	Rotate each shoulder in a slow circular movement; first backwards for 3 circles, and then forwards for 3 circles. Shrug both shoulders up to the ears and drop. Repeat 3 times.
Lower back ache	Poor sitting posture Standing for long periods Lifting Driving	Forward bend Backward bend Spinal twist Cat pose	Clasp the hands in front of the body, round the spine and drop the chin to the chest. Hold the stretch. Now take the palms of the hands and place them in the small of the back. Lift the chest towards the ceiling and slightly raise the chin. This can be done either standing or sitting.
Aching legs and feet	Standing for long periods Poor circulation when seated	Toe and ankle exercises Squatting Leg bend	Flex and point each foot. Rotate the ankles in slow circles, in one direction and then the other.

The problem	Possible work-related causes	Yoga exercises to help	Quick fix
Eye strain	Computer work Poor lighting Driving Tiredness	Eye exercises	Rub the palms of your hands together until you can feel a warmth. Gently place the heel of the palm of each hand over your closed eyes. Feel the warmth of your hands soothe your eyes.
Muscle and joint stiffness	Sitting for long periods Poor posture Driving	Finger and wrist exercises Arm stretch Toe and ankle exercises Squatting Leg bend	Get up and stretch your body with the arms above your head. Give the legs and arms a good shake and go for a quick walk.
Breathing problems	Poor ventilation Panic, anxiety	Breathing exercises Relaxation Chest expansion	With the hands on the diaphragm and the eyes shut, breathe in and out slowly and deeply. Breathe in for 4 counts and out for 4 counts, slow and rhythmically until the breathing and the heart beat slows down.
Repetitive stress injury	Repetitive tasks Keyboard work	Arm stretch Finger and wrist exercises	Flex the wrists upwards and then downwards. Hold the wrist of one hand with the other. Move the fingers as if playing the piano. Repeat with the other hand.

The problem	Possible work-related causes	Yoga exercises to help	Quick fix
Stomach discomfort; heartburn, indigestion, nervous stomach, period pains	Poor posture Nervousness Heavy or rushed lunch	Forward bend (sitting) Knee to forehead	Sitting, bring the knee towards the chest. Keep the back straight and press the knee towards the body. Breathe deeply, feeling the stomach muscles move in and out. Change legs. *Remember, do not do exercises on a full stomach.*
Lethargy, yawning	Boredom Poor ventilation Static position	Breathing exercises Relaxation Meditation Lion pose Rib opening	Take a deep breath through the nose, exhale through the mouth. Repeat several times. If possible, get some fresh air.
Nervous conditions; panic, fear, anger	Deadlines Heavy workloads Crises Insecurity Interviews, presentations	Calming breath Meditation Relaxation	Sit with your eyes closed and your hands in your lap. Breathe slowly and rhythmically. Focus completely on the rise and fall of the breath.

10

Yoga Relief for Travelling

THE TRAUMA OF COMMUTING

Most people will have some form of journey to work. You might walk, drive or take public transport. Unreliable and crammed public transport or traffic jams can result in many people feeling stressed and frazzled even before they get to work. There can be no doubt that this is a bad start to the day! It is so important, however difficult, to try to keep calm in these situations and to conserve your energy for work. More often than not you will have no control over the traffic jam or the bus being late, so letting yourself get wound up is a pointless waste of energy. Here are a few tips to reduce stress when travelling to and from work:

- Give yourself plenty of time to complete your journey, so that if something does delay you, being late and having to rush does not add to your stress. It is tempting to get out of bed at the last possible moment, but it is far better to arrive at work a little early because you have had a smooth journey than to start the day feeling hassled because you were delayed.
- Try to use your journey time to focus your thoughts in preparation for the day. Sit and just concentrate on the rise and fall of the breath. It will be particularly beneficial to

carry out this simple exercise when you feel yourself becoming stressful and anxious, such as while waiting for a delayed bus, when your train has ground to a halt for no apparent reason, or when stuck in a traffic jam. This simple focusing on the breath will calm your body and mind – but be careful not to become too relaxed and fall asleep, and make sure to watch your belongings.

- It might help to absorb yourself in a book, the newspaper or to listen to music on your walkman. This will distract your attention from any problems and stop that frequent 'clock-watching' which will increase your stress levels.

- When you are confronted with a travel problem and feel yourself becoming uptight, be firm and try to put the situation in perspective. Is the fact that you are going to be late for work or late home really a major problem? More often than not it probably isn't, and you should not let yourself over-react to the situation.

DRIVING

Driving is potentially a very stressful activity. Traffic jams, inconsiderate fellow drivers, road works, bad weather conditions and not knowing where you are going can all increase your anxiety levels behind the wheel. Indeed, 'road rage', the term given to anger and aggression in drivers, is recognized as a major problem in many countries. In the United Kingdom the Automobile Association have produced a stress pack for drivers, giving guidance and tips on how to keep road rage at bay.

Drivers also have to concentrate hard for long periods, which can be mentally and physically very tiring. When you are driving, you are in a static position and carrying out a range of repetitive movements: moving the gear stick, pushing the foot pedals, turning the steering wheel, looking in the driver's mirror. You will therefore be prone to the symptoms listed in

Chapter 3 for static and repetitive work. Problems specific to driving may include:

- tense and tender shoulders and upper back from general tension and steering-wheel motion
- stiff neck from looking in the driver's mirror
- backache from an uncomfortable seat
- stiffness and numbness in the buttock area from sitting for long periods
- headaches from concentration and general stress
- strained and sore eyes from peering at the road; this can be aggravated by reflected sunlight, headlights and light reflection off wet roads
- stiff and cramped ankles from operating the pedals
- stiff joints, particularly the knees, from sitting for a long time
- general feeling of lethargy due to lack of fresh air and immobility of the body
- general feeling of restlessness due to confinement of the body

Yoga exercises for drivers

We do not recommend that you attempt to carry out any exercises when you are on the road, even when stationary in a traffic jam or queue, which might in any way impair your concentration. However, there are exercises that you can do when having a break that will greatly relieve the symptoms of driving. These include:

- **Breathing exercises** When you are stuck in a traffic jam and feeling stressful, try just listening to the rise and fall of the breath. This simple exercise will slow your heart rate and keep your stress in check. If you are feeling particularly wound up pull off the road and while sitting quietly carry out the calming breath exercise (page 82) to regulate your breathing. This can also greatly energize and invigorate the body, so deep breathing will also help if you feel yourself becoming drowsy while driving.

- **Yoga exercises for driving breaks** Exercises you might find beneficial when you are taking a break include:

Exercises that can be done in the car (when stationary):
  neck and head roll
  shoulder lifts and rotation
  shoulder opening (space permitting)
  arm stretch (space permitting)
  backwards bend (slightly modified for less space)
  finger and wrist exercises
  ankle and feet exercises
  head and face massage
  buttock raising
  thigh rocking

Standing exercises:
  rib opening
  and any of the others, if you won't feel too silly doing them in a layby or car park!

Other tips for comfortable driving

- **Always take regular breaks when driving long distances** It is tempting to keep on going to reach your destination as soon as possible, but it is important to give yourself a break to stretch your legs, get some fresh air and relax for a few moments. It is dangerous to continue driving if your concentration is impaired in any way, through being tired or uncomfortable. If you take a break, you will be less prone to the physical symptoms mentioned above.

- **Refreshments** Remember always to have something to drink in the car, preferably water, and some energy-giving snacks. Dried fruit or fresh fruit and nuts are preferable to crisps and confectionery. There is a great tendency to eat sweet things in the car out of boredom, but these are of low value nutritionally and can cause an imbalance of energy levels (see Chapter 7).

- **Music** Many people find that playing soothing music calms them down in the car. But do not choose something so relaxing that it makes you feel sleepy!

- **Aromatherapy** You can use aromatherapy oils, placed on a tissue, to freshen the air in your car. Try oils that you find refreshing, such as mandarin or lavender. There are also specific oils available to uplift your spirits, relax you and even help prevent car sickness. Remember that aromatherapy oils can have a very potent effect, so take advice on which ones are suitable, and try to avoid those that are sleep-inducing.

AIR TRAVEL

This is the age of air travel, when people fly from one continent to another for a one-hour meeting! Many businessmen and women will be required to travel by air for their work and it is worth looking at the particular problems that this may create, and what yoga exercises are appropriate.

Like driving, air travel involves the passenger sitting still for long periods. In theory it is possible to stand and stretch your legs, but in practice these opportunities are limited due to lack of space, trolleys being pushed up and down the narrow aisles and having to ask people to get up to let you out. Physical side-effects of flying, particularly for long-haul flights, might be:

- backache
- general stiffness of the joints
- cramped and numb buttocks from sitting for long periods
- swollen ankles from the high altitude

- cold feet from poor circulation and cabin pressure
- general feeling of restlessness from being immobile for long periods

Yoga exercises that can be carried out in a chair and will be particularly helpful in this situation include:
    neck and head roll
    shoulder rotation and shoulder lifts
    shoulder opening
    head to knee (space permitting)
    spinal twist (modified to adapt to space)
    ankle and feet exercises
    finger and wrist exercises
    buttock raising
    thigh rocking

The flight time will also be an ideal opportunity to practise your relaxation and meditation. This will be especially beneficial if you find it hard to sleep on the plane, and the exercises will still leave you feeling relaxed and refreshed.

A few more tips for air travellers

Regular air travellers will be well practised in the art of keeping fresh and comfortable during flight, but it is worth noting the following tips:

- **Dehydration** There is a tendency for the body to become dehydrated during flights, due to the cabin air pressure. Remember to drink plenty of fluids and try to avoid alcohol, which only increases the problem. Skin becomes very dehydrated during long flights, so carry moisturizing lotion if necessary.

- **Ear problems** To combat discomfort and popping in the ears, suck a sweet or chew gum for takeoff and landing. Small yawning motions, or very gently pressing the centre of the ear, can also help the ears to pop gently if they become blocked in flight. If you suffer badly from ear problems during flights, ask your doctor for further advice.

- **Swollen feet and ankles** Feet and ankles often swell in the air. Remember to wear comfortable shoes, or remove them during the flight. Feet can often get cold, especially during night flights, so if removing shoes take a pair of socks (sometimes these are provided).

- **Neck pillows** To increase comfort when sleeping, try an inflatable neck pillow. These take up very little room when deflated and can be easily inflated on the air plane. The pillow gives the neck support at the back and sides and prevents the head from lolling around during sleep.

TRAIN

Travelling by train also involves sitting for long periods, but it is usually easier to get up and stretch your legs. However, for long train journeys, all the exercises suggested for flying will be of benefit and will help you to arrive at your destination feeling fresh and not too stiff.

11

Introduction to the Exercises

Now we come to the most important part of the book – the exercises. So far we have explained how yoga can help you, but now is the time to put it all into practice. We are not asking you to do the headstand in the middle of work, or to split your skirt or trousers trying to get into some impossible position! The exercises are all straightforward and easy to do.

THE SELECTION OF EXERCISES

All the exercises have been chosen because they tackle the specific problems you may experience at work and because they do not require much space or time. They are simple but effective exercises that you will master easily. We are aware that you may not be able to find a place where you can do them on your own, and so we have chosen those that will not draw too much attention to yourself. We have also checked that you can do them all in a variety of work clothes.

A healthy spine is essential to good health, and many of the exercises concentrate on improving the condition of the spine. Our spine can move in four ways: forwards, backwards, sideways and twisting. We include exercises to work the spine in all four directions to maximize the flexibility of the back. Tension builds in the neck and shoulder region in particular, and several exercises work on this area.

The exercises are divided into five sections: breathing, relaxation, meditation, sitting and standing. The breathing exercises come first because good breath control is the basis for all the other exercises. In the sitting exercises, we work through the body from the head and neck to the feet, finishing with eye exercises and the fun lion pose. We have kept the standing exercises simple for the workplace; we start with upward stretches, follow with the standing variation of the forward, backward and sideways bends and twists, and finish with a simple balance. The relaxation and meditation exercises are simple and can be used at work or at home.

The choice of exercises creates a balance of stretches, twists, balances and exercises for mobility of the joints. Add to these the breathing, relaxation and meditation exercises and we have a perfect menu with which to treat the body and the mind and to create a harmonious balance between the two.

How to use this section

There are easy-to-follow instructions for each exercise, with illustrations for extra guidance. We explain the particular benefits of each exercise and give you some teaching tips to help you along your way. Take time to read the instructions and look at the illustrations before you start. At the end of the individual exercises there is a selection of work programmes to help you choose which ones to do each day.

How often to do the exercises

You can do individual exercises throughout the day to help tackle a particular problem, such as the shoulder rotation for tense shoulders, or the breathing exercises to calm you down before a meeting.

But for maximum benefit we recommend that every day you follow the simple ten to fifteen minute programmes given in Chapter 13. These programmes have been carefully designed to exercise and rebalance the whole body in approximately ten minutes. If you can't do them every day, try for at least three times a week. Daily practice will bring about the most benefits. If you think you cannot spare the time, think of all the odd minutes you waste in an average day at work. You just need to find ten minutes to spend on yourself; the benefits will last the whole day and beyond.

Yoga at home/local classes

If you miss your programme at work you may find time to do some exercises in the evening at home or join a local class. We also recommend that you try to find time to keep up your yoga practice at the weekend. At home you may want to try a wider range of yoga exercises. You will have more time, space and privacy, and will be able to wear less restricting clothes, for example, a tracksuit. It will therefore be an ideal opportunity to try out the floor exercises and exercises that need more space and freedom of movement. We list several suitable books under the section on further reading.

The importance of regular practice

You may have been suffering from symptoms of stress for a long time. Do not expect them to disappear overnight after your first yoga session. You might notice small improvements from early on, but the main effect will be cumulative.

Preparing to do the exercises

It is very important to prepare yourself before carrying out your yoga programme, and to pay attention to creating the right environment within which to do your daily practice. If you rush into the exercises with work still on your mind or if you are interrupted it will be very hard to get the most from the yoga session.

Everyone will have a different work environment; you may have your own office or work space, or you may share one with a dozen or more other people. Your boss may be down the corridor, or in a different building, or he or she may even be in the same room as you! You may find it virtually impossible to be undisturbed for even the shortest period, or you may work in a quiet environment. Your work routine and your boss may be flexible, allowing you to take ten minutes out to do your exercises, or you may work in a more regimented set-up with specific break times when you have to leave your work station and go to a canteen. You may work behind the scenes or you may be on the front-line, for example, a receptionist or sitting in a showroom in view of clients.

Whatever your particular circumstances are, try to make the best of the situation when it comes to your yoga practice – remember that even if you are exercising in a less-than-ideal environment, it is still better than not doing them at all and you will still feel the benefit.

Finding the right time and place for yoga at work

Find a time to suit you to carry out the programme of exercises, when you know you will not be disturbed. Try to make this a regular time, so it will become part of your daily routine. You may want to do the exercises during your lunch, coffee or tea break, but for maximum effect, they should not be done on a full stomach. It is a general rule that exercise should not be performed until one-and-a-half hours after a meal, because when your stomach is digesting food you may feel discomfort or nausea, however gentle the exercise. In particular, some of the forward bends and other movements may put pressure on the abdominal area and cause discomfort.

Try to choose a time when the risk of interruption or distraction will be minimized. We realize that this might not be easy, but do your best; maybe choose a time when your fellow workers are at lunch, or a time of the day when your workplace is not quite so busy. Perhaps there is an empty meeting room or office you can use. One yoga student even used to sit in the stationery cupboard so she could do her relaxation exercises in peace!

If you have your own work room, put a note on the door to prevent people from disturbing you, divert your telephone or ask that no calls be put through for ten minutes. If you share a work space, tell your colleagues that you are going to do your exercises and ask them not to disturb you. If you have no option but to do your exercises with others working around you, it will be particularly important that you concentrate very hard and try to distance yourself mentally from your work environment. Try to do the exercises facing a wall to minimize the visual distractions. You do not want to do your exercises while looking at a notice board covered with work memos, so put up an inspiring picture or photograph on which to focus, if appropriate.

If you share a work space, tell your colleagues what you are doing. If you involve them, they are less likely to tease you. Try not to be self-conscious – when they see how much better you feel, they will probably want to join in too! You may even want to try group yoga sessions at work. It will be easier to keep up your daily practice if you have others to encourage you.

If several of you do daily yoga, you might be able to persuade your organization to set aside an unused room for your practice. This would be ideal as it would remove you from your workplace with its noise and distraction and provide you with a quiet retreat where you could also enjoy a few minutes' undisturbed relaxation during the day.

What to wear

Yoga is best done in loose clothing. Tight clothes will restrict movement and may cause discomfort. It would be ideal if you could slip into a T-shirt before you carry out your ten-minute programme. If this is not possible, do not worry – you will still be able to do the exercises. For the greatest comfort and freedom of movement, remove your jacket, loosen your tie and collar and remove your belt.

It is possible to do the exercises in a skirt, but the leg bend, knee to forehead exercise and the dancer balance may be difficult to do properly in a very tight or very long skirt. Glasses should be removed in case they slip off. The eye exercises should not be done if you are wearing contact lenses.

Yoga is traditionally done in bare feet. This is for many reasons: to exercise the feet; to work on the many reflexology zones; to let the feet breathe; to prevent slipping and to assist balance. It would be ideal if you could do your yoga practice barefoot, but this may cause problems, especially if you are wearing tights or are in a shared work space! Always remember, however, to remove your shoes. If you are wearing heels you will not get the full benefit from the exercises.

If you cannot do it at work, try doing yoga barefoot at home. You will find out how good it feels.

Using your chair

Many of the exercises are designed to be done in your chair. This is to make it easier for you to do the exercises throughout the day. The ideal chair would be one with no arms and no wheels. If you only have access to a chair with wheels, take particular care; make sure that the chair is as secure as possible and place your feet firmly on the floor during the exercises to prevent it moving. If the floor is a surface other than carpet, please be extra careful when doing the exercises using a chair with wheels.

Getting into the right frame of mind

Take time to prepare yourself before starting the exercises. Try to allow a few seconds to close your eyes and to inhale and exhale rhythmically, focusing on the breath. This will calm you down and focus your mind before you start. Try to clear your mind of all thoughts about your work. If you are doing your exercises in a noisy environment try very hard just to concentrate on your breath and on yourself and to remove yourself mentally from your workplace.

It will take some time before you are able to quickly clear your mind and stop thinking about work, but it will be easier each time you practise. As mentioned above, it may help if you focus on a picture that you find inspiring or calming, for example, a poster of beautiful scenery.

Try not to rush through the exercises. Spend a few seconds between each to focus on the breath again.

When you are doing the exercises focus on yourself. At work you are always thinking in terms of other people, but when you are doing the exercises it is time for you to think of yourself only.

Listen to your body and make a mental note of how you feel before the exercises and how you feel afterwards. Do you feel different each time you carry out your programme?

GENERAL TIPS

1 Check your posture before starting every exercise. Your back, neck and head should be in a straight line and your stomach muscles held in. This quick posture check will ensure that you do the exercises correctly. Check also that your shoulders are relaxed. If you are carrying tension in the shoulders, you restrict your freedom of movement.

2 When using the chair, make sure your feet are placed firmly on the floor for stability.

3 Breathe in and out through your nose while doing all the exercises. This is fundamental for yoga.

4 Never bounce the body while in a yoga position. Bouncing causes quick contractions of the stretched muscle and can cause injury.

5 If the yoga position is uncomfortable, breathe deeply in and out and try to relax into the stretch.

6 Listen to your body. If any position is too uncomfortable do not force yourself to hold it.

7 Keep an old tie or belt at work. This can be used to assist you with some of the exercises.

Medical note

The exercises in this book are not strenuous. But if you should suffer from high blood pressure, heart complaints, respiratory problems or back injuries, or if you are pregnant or recovering from any operation or chronic illness, please check with your doctor before commencing any form of exercise.

12

The Exercises

LIST OF EXERCISES

Standing exercises p. 125

QUICK POSTURE CHECK

Correct body alignment is essential to yoga, and all the exercises require you to start with this quick posture check. This is the starting point for every yoga exercise.

- back, neck and head should be in a straight line (no arched back, no jutting chin); feel tall and an upward pull of the spine
- the shoulders should be down and relaxed
- the buttocks should be very slightly tucked under
- the stomach muscles should be held firm (not gripped)

Try to remember to carry out this simple check a few times a day. Just think to yourself: back, neck and head in a straight line, shoulders relaxed, buttocks down and stomach in. By doing this you will gradually begin to increase your awareness of your posture and re-educate the body to adopt the correct alignment. This will in turn help to reduce backache and other posture-related aches and pains, and will make you look more poised and confident.

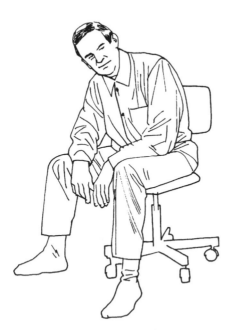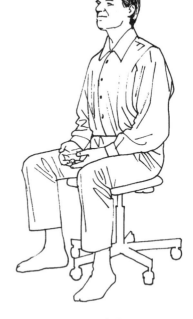

Figure 1   Incorrect sitting posture   *Figure 2   Correct sitting posture*

BREATHING EXERCISES

You might well ask: 'Why breathing exercises? Haven't I been breathing all my life?' Of course you have, but maybe not in a way to obtain the maximum benefit for your body. Did you know that the average person only uses one-fifth of his/her lung capacity? Stop breathing, and your life ends. You can exist for a few days without liquid and a few weeks without food, but without air you would only last a few minutes. The oxygen in air is the life source for your body – just think how wonderful you might feel if you used more of your lung capacity!

The body reacts quickly to a lack of oxygen. Have you ever wondered why you yawn while at work or why you feel so invigorated when you walk in the fresh air of the countryside? When you yawn, it is generally a signal that your body is striving for more oxygen to enter the bloodstream. This could either be because you are very tired and the body needs extra oxygen to continue to perform, or because there is a lack of fresh air in your workplace. When you are short of breath after physical exertion, you will feel exhausted because the body is deprived of oxygen. Similarly, people suffering from respiratory problems, such as asthma, will feel depleted of energy. Breathing brings us energy, and the deeper we breathe the more we will energize our bodies.

We breathe in oxygen to energize the body cells and we breathe out carbon dioxide to remove toxins from the body cells. When we breathe in deeply, we nourish all the vital parts of our body; energy is sent, via the bloodstream, to the vital organs, to the glands and to our nerve centres. The correct way to breathe is through the nose with its built-in filter, not through your mouth. Correct breathing filters out germs and can help prevent colds and sore throats.

Let us pause here to consider the body's breathing apparatus. When we breathe, we draw in air through our nasal passages. It passes down our windpipe and through our bronchial tubes into the millions of small air spaces that make up the lungs. The blood flows through these tiny air cells and becomes oxygenated. It is then pumped back through the heart to the whole body, supplying every part with energy. The diaphragm, a large flat muscle that divides the area of the chest from the abdomen draws the air into the lungs. When it flattens, it increases the size of the lungs and the air rushes in; when it relaxes it causes the lungs to contract and expel the air.

Yoga teaching often refers to four types of breathing; high, mid, low and complete. High breathing is when only the upper portion of the lung is used and the collar bone rises. This breathing is very common, but is thought to be the worst type because a large amount of energy is expended, but very little air is taken into the lungs.

Mid breathing is when the middle portion of the lungs is used and the chest expands slightly sideways as well as upwards. Low breathing is preferable to high and mid breathing. It is sometimes referred to as abdominal breathing and it results in a larger intake of air. The ideal breath would be one that uses all parts of the lungs and enables the largest intake of air, and this is referred to as full or complete breathing.

Yoga breathing is complete breathing, which means we fill our lungs with the maximum amount of air and provide our bodies with the maximum amount of energy. By doing the yoga breathing exercises we will feel invigorated as if we have been walking in the fresh air.

Breathing corresponds to our emotions. If you are excited or frightened your breathing rate will accelerate and the breath will become more shallow. If you are relaxed and calm, your breathing rate will reflect this as in sleep when the breathing is usually deep and slow. But this situation works vice versa. By controlling our breathing we can affect our emotions. Regulated breathing can be a powerful stress-management tool.

Take a moment now to listen to your breathing. Inhale and feel your abdomen wall expand outwards; exhale and feel it contract back towards your spine. Put your hands on your abdomen wall and breathe slowly and deeply through your nose. Feel the abdomen move outwards and inwards. Close your eyes for a moment and just listen to your breathing. Even a few minutes of this slow rhythmical breathing brings about a calmness and a peace of mind.

Let us now practise the specific breathing exercises. These exercises are very powerful and if at any time you feel light-headed, stop immediately and breathe normally.

1 The full breath exercise

The full breath combines low, mid and high breathing all in one. It uses all the breathing apparatus and the maximum amount of benefit is obtained for the minimum expenditure of energy. The full breath, if practised regularly, is also thought to increase your immunity to colds and bronchial and respiratory problems. This exercise will regulate the breath and quickly calm and relax you. The deep breaths will also fill you with energy and nourish the body.

Take time to become familiar with the full breath as it forms the basis for the other breathing exercises mentioned in this section. Try it at periods throughout the day.

1 Sit comfortably in a chair with your back, neck and head in a straight line. You can keep your eyes open or closed, whatever feels more comfortable for you. Place the feet firmly on the floor.
2 Place the hands on your abdomen wall as in *figure 3*.
3 Slowly inhale through your nose. Firstly feel the abdomen wall expand naturally as the breath starts, and secondly feel the breath move up through your mid-chest and feel the ribs expand sideways and backwards. Finally, feel the breath rise to the upper chest. All three movements should be done within the one full breath. Do not raise your shoulders because this will prevent you from using your full lung capacity.
4 Slowly exhale, feeling the upper chest and ribs return to

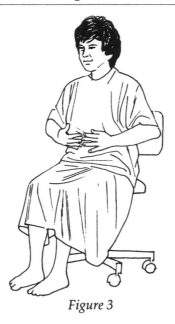

Figure 3

position and the abdominal wall relax and contract back towards your spine.

5 Repeat the full breath for a few times.
6 Now slowly inhale with the full breath to a count of three to five seconds.
7 Exhale slowly to a count of three to five seconds.
8 Repeat three to five times with the counting.

Tip: Start by counting for only three seconds and when you feel ready build up to five seconds. Remember to always breathe through the nose only and to keep your shoulders relaxed. Do not think of the breath as three separate movements but as one continuous movement through the abdomen, ribs and upper chest. This will become easier with practice. If you feel light-headed at any time during the exercise, stop immediately and breathe normally. Only repeat the full breath for a few times and then relax; it is a very powerful exercise and can make you slightly dizzy if you repeat it too often without a break.

2 Basic breathing exercises

Try these simple exercises which are all variations on the full breath exercise above. Start each exercise sitting comfortably with the back straight unless otherwise stated. Always breathe through the nose unless otherwise stated. Keep the eyes open or closed, whatever you prefer. If you experience any dizziness in any of the exercises, stop immediately and breathe normally.

Exercise 1
1 Sit with the arms loose at your sides (*figure 4*). Inhale with the full breath and lift the arms straight to the sides and above your head with the fingers touching (*figure 5*).

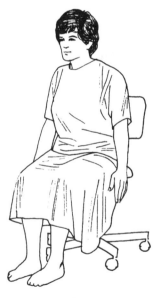

Figure 4

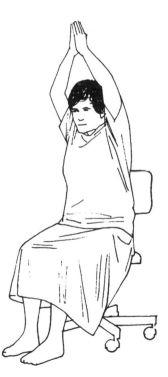

Figure 5

2 Hold the breath for two to three seconds.
3 Exhale slowly and lower the hands to the sides of the body.
4 Relax.
5 Repeat up to three times.

Exercise 2
1 Sit with the arms straight in front of you at shoulder level, palms facing down (*figure 6*). This exercise can also be done standing.
2 Inhale with the full breath and swing the arms to the sides slightly behind your shoulders (*figure 7*).
3 Exhale slowly and return the arms to in front of you.
4 Relax.
5 Repeat up to 3 times.

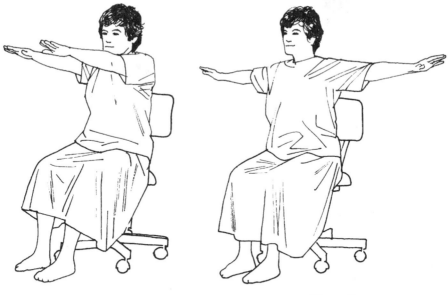

Figure 6   *Figure 7*

Exercise 3
1 Stand or sit straight with the arms bent and the hands in front of your chest (*figure 8*).

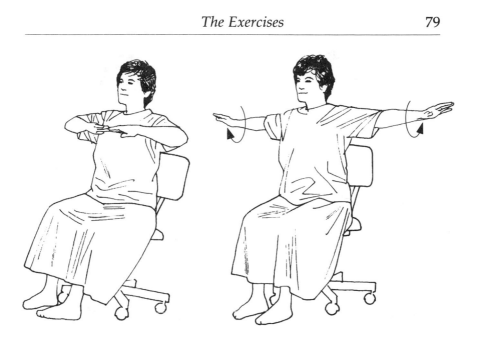

Figure 8   Figure 9

2 Inhale with the full breath and take the arms to the sides at shoulder level (*figure 9*).
3 Hold the breath and rotate the arms for three backwards circles.
4 Exhale vigorously and return the hands to the chest.
5 Repeat three times.
6 Relax.

Exercise 4
1 Inhale with the full breath and tense every muscle in your body (*figure 10*).
2 Hold the breath and tension for three seconds.
3 Exhale through the mouth and let all the muscles relax and the arms hand free at your side (*figure 11*).
4 Repeat three times.

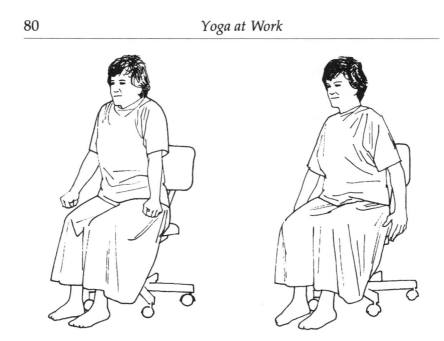

Figure 10   Figure 11

Exercise 5
This is an exercise to relieve blocked nasal passages.
1 Inhale in three or four sniffing motions. Do not exhale in between but do as one inhalation.
2 Exhale slowly.
3 Repeat three times.

3 Alternate nostril breathing

Preparation for alternate nostril breathing
This exercise will also help unblock the nasal passages and is a good preparation for alternate nostril breathing.

1 Close one nostril with the first and middle finger, and with a sniffing action take five to ten short breaths through the open nostril. Breathe normally.
2 Repeat with the other nostril.

Alternate nostril breathing

This exercise shows how to use alternate nostril breathing. This breathing technique helps unblock the nostrils and ease breathing difficulties. It is also a powerful cleansing and re-energizing exercise, which will leave you feeling clear-headed and calm.

Using the right hand, practise the position of the hand for this exercise. Use the thumb to close the right nostril and the ring finger to close the left nostril. The two middle fingers should rest on the forehead, between the eyebrows. Practise closing each nostril until you feel comfortable with the position of the fingers.

1 Block the right nostril with the thumb of the right hand and inhale through the left nostril for the count of three (*figure 12*).
2 Block the left nostril with the ring finger and exhale through the right nostril for the count of three (*figure 13*).
3 Keep the left nostril blocked, and inhale through the right nostril for the count of three.
4 Block the right nostril and exhale through the left nostril for the count of three.

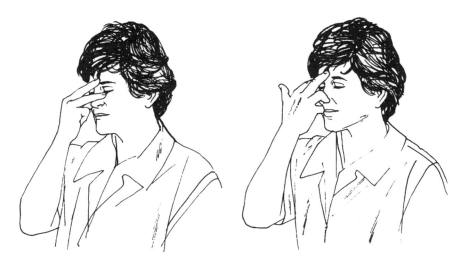

Figure 12   *Figure 13*

This sequence (1–4) makes up one round of alternate nostril breathing. Repeat for at least three rounds, building up to five as you become more practised at the technique.

4 Full breath with breath retention

Now try this exercise which increases control of the lungs.

1 Sit comfortably with your back, neck and head in a straight line and the eyes closed.
2 Put your hands on your abdomen wall, or, if you prefer, rest them in your lap.
3 Inhale with the full breath slowly for a count of three to five seconds.
4 Hold the breath for a count of three to five seconds.
5 Exhale slowly for a count of three to five seconds.
6 Repeat three to five times.

Tip: Start with three seconds and build up to five seconds after practice. Try not to raise the shoulders when you hold the breath as this reduces your lung capacity. Do not let the exhalation gush out; try to control it.

5 The calming breath

To calm yourself quickly, try this simple and effective exercise. Breathe slowly, focusing on the breath, and make the out breath twice as long as the in breath. For example, breathe in for two counts and out for four, or in for three and out for six. This will automatically calm you down, reduce your heart rate and release any tension. You can do it at any time during the day; after a stressful telephone call or confrontation, before a meeting or interview. No one will even know you are doing it!

RELAXATION EXERCISES

Relaxation is a much spoken about, but little understood, state of being. We often confuse relaxation with rest, but the two are not necessarily synonymous. To rest is to abstain from exertion and action, but that does not automatically mean freedom from tension. Relaxation is a conscious letting go of tension, an art to be studied and mastered.

The society in which we live is beset with tensions, and this is particularly true of the busy workplace. It is therefore even more important to induce complete physical, mental and emotional relaxation and so create a one-pointedness in our mind.

Ideally, relaxation should be practised whilst lying flat on the floor so that you are aware of your tension points from head to toe. Obviously, this cannot be done at work, so we suggest practising at home. The room should be well-ventilated and warm, or you can cover yourself with a blanket. There should be no noise, such as the television or radio, but you can, if you wish, use soothing music. It should be unobtrusive and gentle. There are many tapes available on the market for the purpose of relaxation.

Relaxation can also be carried out successfully in a chair and so you can practise it in the office or workplace. It would be ideal if you could do your relaxation alone in a quiet room; perhaps in an unused office or meeting room. If not, you can do it at work, but if there is background noise such as voices and ringing phones it will make it harder for you to cut yourself off totally and fully relax. If you have your own office or work room, put a 'Do not disturb' notice on your door and remember to divert your phone calls for the duration of your relaxation session.

A few minutes' conscious relaxation can have a very beneficial effect. You can experience a feeling of complete refreshment and a new feeling of awareness. Your mind will become clear and you will feel able to tackle your problems in a more objective manner. When mastered, the art of relaxation can bring joy, an increased efficiency, improved power of concentration and an ability to relate well to other people, your family and your work colleagues. If practised regularly it can completely reshape your outlook on life and put all things into perspective.

In Western society, we often rush for the tranquillizers or for substitutes such as alcohol when we feel stressed, but when the effects wear off the problem remains. In the East, it was realized centuries ago that peace of mind could only be achieved from within and not from external sources. You must first become aware of the physical, mental and emotional tensions affecting you and then tackle them at source.

Relaxation exercise

This exercise should take approximately five to ten minutes to do, depending on the amount of time you can spare. It will be beneficial, if you have the time, to spend longer in the deep relaxation state after you have carried out the auto-suggestions.

1 Sit comfortably in your chair with your hands resting in your lap or on your thighs. Close your eyes and inhale and exhale slowly and gently. Listen to your in-going and out-going breath. Try to shut everything else out of your mind.
2 Now be aware of your body. Tell it to relax, relax, relax. Repeat this to yourself a few times. A feeling of calmness will gradually be induced in your whole body. Difficult perhaps at first, but the more you persist and the less you worry about it, the easier it will become.
3 Now give auto-suggestions to the different parts of your body from head to foot. Working your way through the body, say the following auto-suggestions three times each to yourself:

I am relaxing my feet × 3
I am relaxing my legs × 3
I am relaxing my thighs × 3

I am relaxing my hips × 3
I am relaxing my stomach × 3
I am relaxing my chest × 3
I am relaxing my fingers × 3
I am relaxing my hands × 3
I am relaxing my wrists × 3
I am relaxing my lower arms × 3
I am relaxing my elbows × 3
I am relaxing my upper arms × 3
I am relaxing my shoulders × 3
I am relaxing my neck × 3
I am relaxing my eyes × 3
I am relaxing my cheeks × 3
I am relaxing my mouth × 3
I am relaxing my head × 3
I am relaxing my upper body and shoulders × 3
I am relaxing my spine and whole back × 3
I am relaxing my whole body × 3

While giving these auto-suggestions to the different parts of your body, visualize them and induce the feeling of relaxation and letting go in the particular body part. Be aware of what is happening. At first perhaps the mind will wander. Don't worry – this is quite natural. Persevere and practice will bring its reward.

4 Stay in this relaxed state for as long is comfortable and possible.

5 When you are ready, slowly bring the mind back to focus on the breathing and open your eyes.

Tip: After you have relaxed your body by carrying out the auto-suggestions try the following visualization. Think of a beautiful and serene place, maybe somewhere you have been before and which you have loved, for example, a beach, a mountain, a forest, a lake, a garden or any place you find inspiring. Imagine you are in this beautiful place. The mind will wander, but just let these thoughts pass through your mind and then refocus on your scene. Try to feel that you are really there; smell the air, feel the sun on your body and just absorb yourself in the scene. Always come out of relaxation very slowly and sit calmly for a while to readjust to your physical surroundings.

As you become practised at the basic relaxation technique, you will be able to miss, or carry out an abridged version of, the auto-suggestions and go straight into your visualization and start exploring your imagination.

MEDITATION EXERCISES

Why meditate?

The practice of meditation is greatly beneficial; it focuses the mind, clears the senses and relaxes the body. After meditation you will feel revitalized and calm. You will be able to return to your work with increased efficiency, energy and enthusiasm. People speak of how meditation is a journey within yourself; it is a journey that will tap sources of energy and creativity and which will leave you feeling 'centred'. The practice of regular meditation is a powerful tool to de-stress yourself.

Meditation can provide you with answers to your problems, because in silence and with a calm mind, answers will often emerge. The more you meditate the deeper you will be able to go into yourself and experience inner peace, love, beauty and detachment.

Your physical body can also benefit from the practice. Many ailments are psychosomatic and some people find that meditation can have a healing effect.

How to meditate

Meditation is a skill that has to be mastered. There are many different methods and if you wish to pursue any of these you should attend a class or refer to the literature that is available (see the further reading section).

Here, however, we include some very simple meditation exercises that can be mastered easily and that will only take a few minutes each day. The concept behind meditation is that we try to structure our thinking processes until we get control of our thoughts and are able to still our mind. Many techniques for meditation involve focusing on an object – a flower, a sound, an appealing word or a picture – we eventually get lost in it and become one with it. As this happens, time will cease to exist and we will live in the present. The minute we pause to analyse what is happening, we cease to meditate and we are back in our conscious state.

Occasionally we will remember where we have been and we will want to return. People often relate how they experience clear light, peace and serenity during their meditation.

Imagination helps you to meditate, and for that reason we use visualization and guided meditation. Working without a guide or teacher makes meditation a little harder to master; you will have to be disciplined and use will-power.

The use of counting is very beneficial when learning how to meditate. You can listen to the ticking of a clock or a metronome. The best method, however, is to listen to your heartbeat as in this way you will become familiar with the individual rhythm of your body.

Some simple meditation techniques

Sit in a comfortable chair or sofa with your hands hanging loose at your sides or placed on your lap. Hold your head straight, and as in the relaxation technique go through each part of your body and tell it to relax. You may well be surprised at the amount of tension you are actually carrying in your body. Again, it is important that you try to find a quiet place to carry out these exercises.

Below are some techniques to help you start to meditate.

1 **Third eye meditation.** In yoga the area between your two eyes is referred to as the third eye. Lift your eyes slightly upwards and try and focus on this area for a few seconds. Now close your eyes and continue to concentrate on this area. Try to repeat this regularly every day for one week for up to ten to fifteen minutes if possible. If you feel any dizziness or eye strain stop at once and open the eyes.

2 **Television screen visualization.** Visualize a television screen. Imagine that your thoughts are images being projected onto this screen, and as each thought is projected, turn the television off. As you repeat this there will be less and less thoughts and the mind will become quieter. The aim of this exercise is eventually to have a blank television screen.

3 **Beautiful scene visualization.** It is good to begin with a scene that is familiar to you and that is associated with happy experiences, for example, a past holiday destination. Try to imagine yourself at this place and let the beauty fill you with serenity and uplift you.

4 **Counting meditation.** Now begin to concentrate on your breathing. Breathe in and out, in and out, slowly and gently. Now, breathe in slowly for the count of three, 1-2-3 and exhale 1-2-3. Keep this rhythm of breathing; inhale for 1-2-3, exhale for 1-2-3.

The following is a meditation that you might want to practise at home.

5 **Candle-gazing meditation.** This is a most beneficial technique because you lose yourself in the flickering of the candle flame and it brings comfort to your whole body. Gaze at the candle flame and when you are ready close your eyes. When you close your eyes try to retain the image of the flame and focus on this.

Remember to observe how you feel before and after meditation and to monitor your progress. If you are worried about time-keeping, you could ask a friend to come and rouse you after a certain time. Most people will find they naturally come out of the meditation. As you are sitting, there should be little danger of you falling asleep, especially if you keep concentrating on the breath.

Give yourself time to come out of the meditation. Open your eyes slowly and adjust your senses. Observe how you feel afterwards. How did you feel before? Is there a difference?

Do not be impatient if you find it hard to stop your mind wandering at first. This is perfectly natural. The more you practise, the easier it will become.

THE SITTING EXERCISES

1 Neck and Head Roll

FOR: Stiffness and tension in the neck and shoulders.

BENEFITS: Increases mobility of the neck and eases tension and stiffness in the neck and shoulders.

Exercise
1 Sit comfortably in your chair, with the neck, back and head in a straight line. Place the feet firmly on the floor. Rest your hands in your lap. Keep your eyes open throughout the exercise to prevent dizziness.
2 Drop your chin gently towards the chest.
3 Moving the head in a circular motion, gently rotate your chin towards your right shoulder.
4 Continue the circle with the chin lifting towards the ceiling and the head tilting slightly backwards.
5 Rotate the head towards the left and gently drop your chin towards your left shoulder.
6 Move the head to the centre again with your chin resting on your chest.
7 Repeat twice more in this direction (three times in total) and three more times to the left.

Tip: If you have acute muscle tenderness, this exercise may be painful and you should perhaps wait until the situation improves. If you have restricted neck movements due to past injury, you may not find this exercise very easy to do. Do not attempt to force any movement; gentle persistence will probably increase your mobility.

Be very careful when tilting the head backwards, and only tilt it as far as is comfortable. Do not let the head fall back, as

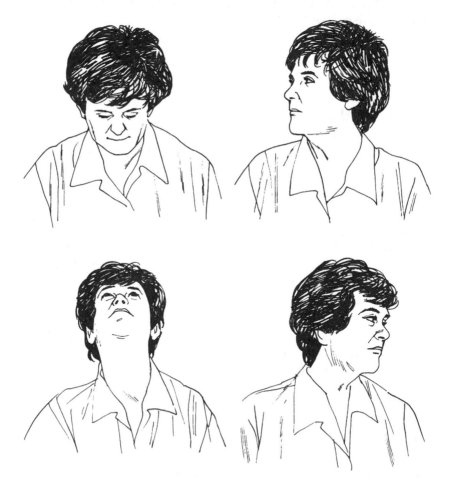

Figure 14

this can jar the neck. Keep the movement smooth. Do not worry if you feel grinding or grating noises in your neck (unless these are associated with pain, in which case you should stop immediately).

If you are prone to dizziness, make sure you do this exercise very slowly. If you feel dizzy at any time, stop immediately and put your head between your knees until you recover.

2 Shoulder Rotation and Shoulder Lifts

FOR: Tense and tender shoulders and upper back.

BENEFITS: Releases the tension that gathers in the shoulder and upper back region. If done regularly throughout the day, this exercise can help prevent shoulder tension build up.

Exercise
1 Sit comfortably and slightly forward in your chair with your back, neck and head in a straight line. Place your feet firmly on the floor, slightly apart. Your arms should be relaxed at your sides. Breathe normally throughout the exercise.
2 Rotate your left shoulder in a slow backwards circle (*figure 15*). Try to brush your ear with your shoulder as you circle, but do not move the head towards the shoulder – that is cheating! Do this slowly three times. Repeat at a faster speed three times.
3 Still using your left shoulder, repeat, this time circling forward: three times slowly and three times a little faster.
4 Repeat the whole sequence with your right shoulder, three slow and three faster backward circles, and three slow and three faster forward circles.
5 Using both shoulders together, rotate for three slow and three fast backward circles. Repeat again in the forwards direction.

Now try the shoulder lifts. This exercise releases all the tension from the shoulders.

1 Lift your right shoulder to your ear, breathing in as you do so.
2 Drop the shoulder back down releasing all the tension, and breathe out, making a slight hissing sound through the mouth.
3 Repeat three times with the right shoulder, and three times with the left shoulder.
4 Repeat three times with both shoulders together.

Tip: If your shoulders are very tender, do the shoulder rotations very gently to start with. As the shoulders loosen up you can then build up to the faster circles. When working one shoulder only, remember to keep the other shoulder relaxed and still.

If you have any neck or shoulder pain or are suffering from any injury in that area, please be very gentle and cautious when carrying out these exercises. Be particularly careful with

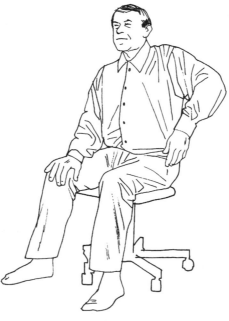

Figure 15

the shoulder lifts and only make small movements to assist the mobility of your shoulder joints.

3 Shoulder and Arm Rotation

FOR: Shoulder and upper back tension.

BENEFITS: Mobilizes the shoulder blades and releases tension in the shoulder region and upper back.

Exercise
1 Sit comfortably with your back, neck and head in a straight line. Place your feet firmly on the floor. Breathe normally throughout the exercise.
2 Place your fingertips on your shoulders and raise your elbows to the side of your body.
3 Keeping your fingertips on your shoulders rotate the elbows in a backwards circle (*figure 16*). Start by bringing the elbows to meet together in front of the chest, part them, lift them up and circle backwards. Repeat for three times altogether.
4 Now repeat in the other direction for three forward circles. This time let the elbows meet in front of your face, drop them, part and continue the forward circles.
5 Drop the arms and give the shoulders a shake to relax.

Tip: Remember to keep the fingers on the shoulders throughout this exercise. Let the shoulders rotate naturally with the movement of the elbows. If the shoulders are very tender, start with very small rotations and do not raise the elbows too high. Keep the head facing straight ahead throughout this exercise.

4 Arm Stretch

FOR: Stiffness in the arm joints and cramped arm muscles and tendons.

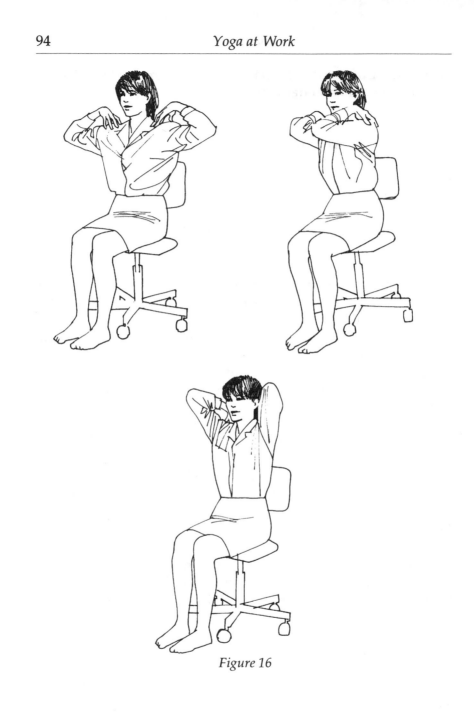

Figure 16

BENEFITS: Mobilizes the elbow joints and stretches the arms tendons which are contracted during keyboard and other desk work.

Exercise
1 Sit comfortably with the back, neck and head in a straight line. Place the feet firmly on the floor. Breathe normally throughout the exercise.
2 Place the fingers on the shoulders and lift the elbows in front of the body to shoulder level (*figure 17*).
3 Keeping the elbows raised, unfold the arms to a straightened position with the hands outstretched, palms upwards (*figure 18*).
4 Bend the arms again, returning the fingers to the shoulders.
5 Repeat the movement three to five times.

Try these two variations of the exercise.

Sideways arm stretch: Repeat the exercise, this time stretching the arms to side of the body at shoulder height (*figure 19*).

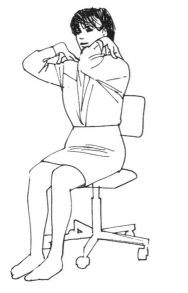

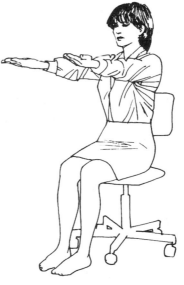

Figure 17   *Figure 18*

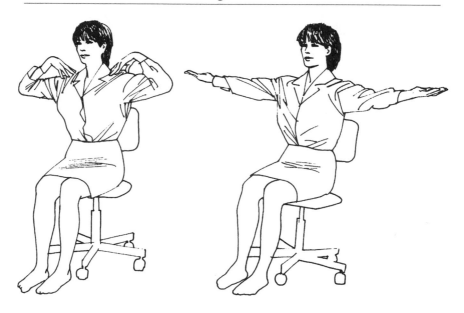

Figure 19

Upwards arm stretch: Repeat the exercise, starting with the elbows at the side of the body and reach the arms above the head shoulder-width apart (*figure 20*).

Tip: Keep the shoulders relaxed. If you raise them the movement will be restricted. For the forwards and sideways arm stretches, keep the elbows at shoulder height throughout the exercise. If the elbows drop, the stretch is not so effective.

5 Finger and Wrist Exercises

FOR: Stiffness, cramp and tenderness in the wrists and fingers.

BENEFITS: Exercises the many tendons in the wrists and fingers and eases stiffness of the wrist and finger joints caused by keyboard work or other repetitive tasks.

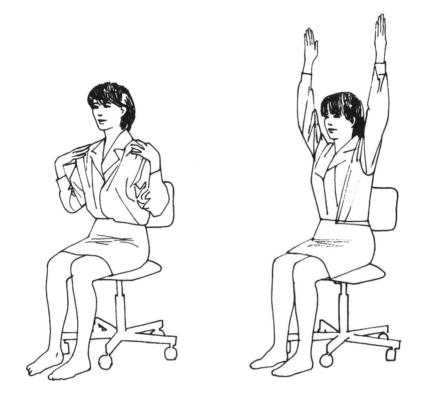

Figure 20

If carried out regularly, this set of exercises can help reduce the risk of repetitive stress injury. These exercises are also known to help to relieve the symptoms of rheumatism in the hands.

Exercise 1
1 Sit comfortably with your back, neck and head in a straight line. Place the feet firmly on the floor.
2 Hold the arms outstretched in front of the body at shoulder level with the palms facing downwards.

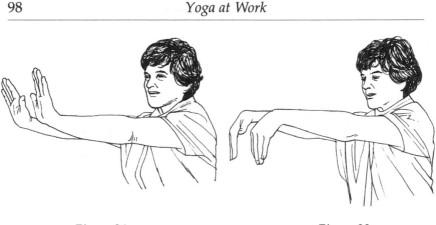

Figure 21   *Figure 22*

3 Flex the wrists and lift the palms to face the opposite wall (*figure 21*).
4 Return the palms to the original position, facing downwards, and then flex the wrists downwards so the palms face towards the body (*figure 22*).
5 Do this movement with the hands moving alternately, one flexed upwards, the other downwards for a few seconds, and then repeat six times with both hands together. Remember to keep the arms straight throughout.

Exercise 2
1 Remain seated as before.
2 With the arms still outstretched, make a fist with the hands placing the thumb in the palm of the hand, under the fingers (*figure 23*).
3 Rotate the wrist three times in an inward circle, and three times in an outward circle.
4 Release the hands and shake the fingers and wrists to release tension.

Exercise 3
1 Remain seated as before.
2 Clench the hands in a fist and bring the hands to the chest (*figure 24*).

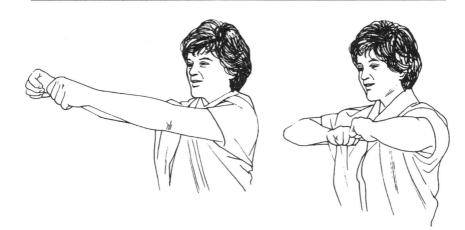

Figure 23   Figure 24

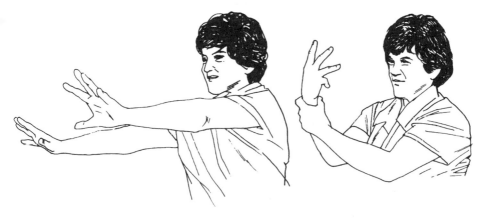

Figure 25   Figure 26

3 In one movement, outstretch the arms forwards at shoulder level and shoot the fingers out (*figure 25*).
4 Return the hands to the chest and clench the fists. Repeat three times.

Exercise 4
1 Still sitting, hold one wrist with the other hand for support.
2 Move all the fingers of the free hand separately as if playing the piano and relax them (*figure 26*).
3 Now separate the fingers making a space between them and relax them.
4 Tense the fingers like a bird's claw and relax them.
5 Shake the hand to release tension and repeat with the other hand.

Tip: In exercises 1–3, keep the arms at shoulder level. Keep the shoulders relaxed at all times and try not to strain the neck. If done regularly, this exercise can help prevent RSI. However, if you are actually suffering from an RSI injury or have had a broken wrist or similar problem, check with your doctor before carrying out any wrist and finger exercises.

6 Head to Knee

FOR: Stiffness in the back region and backache.

BENEFITS: Increases the flexibility of the spine by stretching the back muscles and ligaments. This exercise also eases tension and stiffness in the back region, helps to improve posture and may relieve certain types of lower backache. Improved mobility of the back, especially in older people who may have osteoarthritis of the spine, gives increased confidence in movements of the limbs and of the body as a whole in daily tasks.

The forward bend also nourishes the facial muscles and the brain cells by increasing the blood flow to the head, leaving you feeling refreshed. It also massages the stomach region helping indigestion or discomfort from bloating.

Exercise
1 Sit comfortably with the buttocks to the back of the chair. Place the feet firmly on the floor with the legs hip-distance

apart. Keep the eyes open throughout the exercise to prevent dizziness.

2 Extend the arms up towards the ceiling at the side of the head, and with one arm after the other reach for the ceiling. Feel the stretch through the side of the body and actually feel that with each stretch you are becoming two inches taller (*figure 27*).

3 Inhale, and feel an upwards lift through the body to the tip of the head, but remember to keep the shoulders relaxed. Exhale and, keeping the arms at the sides of the head, bend the torso forward with the chest moving towards the knee. As you bend forward the arms should relax down towards the ankles and floor (*figure 28*).

4 Relax into the position, bending only as far as is comfortable. Feel the pull of gravity increase the stretch. Breathe naturally as you hold the stretch for five to ten seconds.

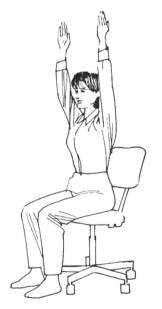

Figure 27

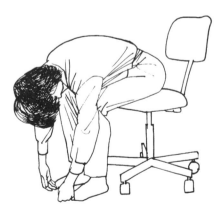

Figure 28

5 Now roll slowly up the spine, inhaling as you do so, to
return to the upright sitting position. Start from the base of
the spine and roll up one vertebra at a time with the head
returning to position last of all. Leave the arms relaxed at
your sides.

Tip: Many people may not get very far with this exercise at
first. Movements must be slow, smooth and deliberate. If resistance in the back stops movement forwards *do not* attempt to
force the position by quick or jerky movements. Instead, hold
the position in which you can feel the resistance for about five
seconds with arms outstretched, allowing gravity to impose a
steady gentle pull downwards on the trunk. In time there will
be improvement in the range of forward movement, although
older people with very stiff backs may never be able to achieve
the full position.

People with acute prolapsed intervertebral discs, or with
acute painful spasm of the back muscles, should *not* attempt
this exercise; however, when the acute stages are over, forward
bends, such as in this exercise, may be very useful in restoring
flexibility and better co-ordination of spinal movements *provided that* such exercises are done gently and with due care at
first.

Care must be taken to keep the spine as straight as possible,
allowing bending only at the lower lumbar area where the
stresses and strains of bending are least likely to cause any
problems. A continual active headward stretching of the whole
body during all stages of the exercises will help to keep the
back straight.

7 Backwards Bend

FOR: Backache, shoulder tension and stiffness in the whole
back region.

BENEFITS: Increases the mobility of the back and relieves

backache and shoulder tension caused by sitting stooped over a desk or work station.

The back bend is a counter pose to the head to knee or forward bend.

Exercise

1 Sit towards the front of your chair with the back, neck and head in a straight line. Place the feet firmly on the floor with the legs hip-distance apart.
2 Hold the sides of your chair firmly at the side of your hips with the elbows slightly bent. Inhale.
3 Pushing the weight into the hands, bend the torso gently backwards, lifting the chest towards the ceiling (*figure 29*). Exhale as you bend the body. Do not drop the head backwards as this may restrict your breath and jar the neck. Keep the head in line with the back with the face towards the ceiling.

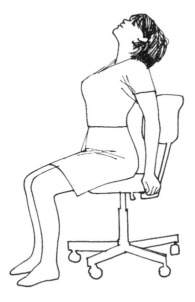

Figure 29

4 Hold the stretch for a few seconds, breathing normally, then inhale and slowly return to the upright position. Exhale.

An alternative position is to straddle the chair so you are facing the back and to hold the back of the chair firmly when leaning backwards. You will not be able to do this if you are wearing a tight-fitting skirt.

Tip: Remember not to drop the head backwards as this will put strain on the neck. Only bend as far as is comfortable. Hold the chair firmly and be particularly careful if you are using a chair with wheels or doing this exercise on a slippery surface.

8 Sideways Bend

FOR: Backache and general stiffness in the torso.

BENEFITS: Increases the flexibility of the spine and stretches all the muscles of the waist and ribs. Like the forward bend, this exercise will bring blood to your head and stimulate the thyroid and parathyroid glands. You will also benefit from some massage of the abdomen area if you remember to keep the stomach muscles firm when bending. After the forward and backwards bend, the sideways bend completes the range of movements.

Exercise
1 Sit comfortably with the back, neck and head in a straight line. Part the feet slightly for stability.
2 Extend the arms to the sides at shoulder level (*figure 30*). With an exhalation of the breath, bend the body to the right side keeping the arms in line with the shoulders as you move (*figure 31*). Bend as far as is comfortable without raising the left buttock off the chair.

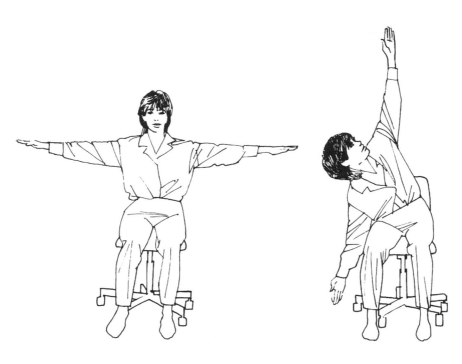

Figure 30   Figure 31

3 Hold the position for three to five seconds, breathing normally. Your right hand should reach towards the floor and the left arm towards the ceiling. Keep your head facing forwards in line with your chest so you do not twist the neck.
4 Return the body to the upright position, inhaling as you do so.
5 Repeat to the left side.

Tip: If the position of the head is causing any neck pain, try looking towards the floor instead.

9 Triangle

FOR: Stiffness in the back.

BENEFITS: Improves your posture by opening the chest and shoulder region, and also works on the stomach muscles and internal organs.

The stretch will work on the hips, waist, sides and armpit areas. The spine is also capable of a twisting motion and doing this movement increases its mobility. The triangle exercise combines the sideways stretch and the twisting movement.

Exercise
1 Sit comfortably with the back, neck and head in a straight line. Place the feet hip-distance apart.
2 Extend the arms to the side of the body at shoulder level.
3 Exhale and twist the body to the left so that the right hand reaches for the left foot (*figure 32*). The left hand will reach up to the ceiling. Keep the head facing the left side, keep it in line with the chest to avoid twisting the neck.
4 Hold this position for three to five seconds, breathing normally. Only twist as far as is comfortable. Your hand may reach the foot, the ankle or the shin. Keep the chest open and feel that you are trying to get the shoulders in line with each other. Look up towards your raised arm, but if this is uncomfortable, look sideways or in any position which does not put strain on the neck.
5 Inhale and return to the upright position.
6 Repeat the twist to the right side with the left hand reaching for the right foot.

Tip: If there is a shortening of muscles on one side, be careful not to over-extend yourself. One side is often more flexible than the other. If you experience any pain in your chest or ringing in the ears, stop at once. Always remember to do both sides to achieve balance. Remember to work slowly and carefully with

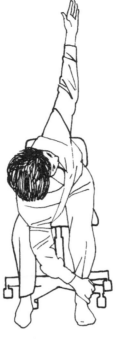

Figure 32

your head and neck and if you feel any discomfort stop straight away.

10 Spinal Twist

FOR: Stiffness of the spine and back muscles.

BENEFITS: Improves flexibility of the spine. It is a very simple exercise that will give you a powerful stretch of the back. It will relieve tension that has built up in your back region, and can be done at any time during the day. The spinal twist will stimulate your kidneys, spleen and liver and reproductive organs. The twist can also help ease constipation and digestive problems as it massages the stomach.

Exercise

1 Sit comfortably with your back, neck and head in a straight line. Keep your feet together.
2 Inhale. Exhale and twist to the left and place both your hands on the back of the chair. Look over your left shoulder at the wall behind and increase the twist, using the back of the chair as leverage (*figure 33*). Keep the left shoulder down and as relaxed as possible. Try to work towards getting the two shoulders in line with each other.
3 Hold the twist, breathing normally, for three to five seconds. Remember to keep both your buttocks firmly on the chair for stability.
4 Inhale and return to the centre position. Repeat the twist to the right side.

Tip: Keep the hips facing the front and firmly in the centre of the chair. Only twist from the waist upwards, not the whole body. Be careful not to strain your neck by looking too far behind.

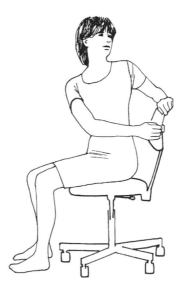

Figure 33

11 Chest Expansion

FOR: Tension in the shoulder and upper back area, and breathing problems.

BENEFITS: Opens the chest and releases tension that gathers in the shoulder and upper back area. This exercise also incorporates a forward bend to stretch the spine and the back muscles, and to bring blood to the head and benefit to the internal organs.

Exercise
1 Sit towards the front of your chair with your back, neck and head in a straight line. Place the feet hip-distance apart. Clasp your hands behind your back with the arms straight.
2 Exhale and bend forwards with the head towards the knee. As you bend raise the clasped hands behind your back towards the ceiling, keeping the arms straight (*figure 34*).

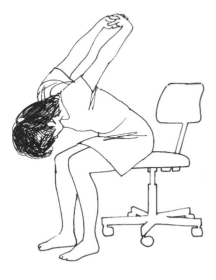
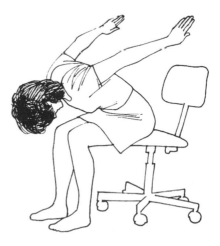

Figure 34   *Figure 35*

3 Bend as far as is comfortable and hold for three to five seconds, breathing normally. Remember to keep those arms straight, if possible.
4 Inhale and roll up the spine returning to the upright position. Repeat once more.
5 Do the backward bend (Exercise 7) as a counter-stretch for this exercise.

Alternative arm position: If you have a shoulder problem or find the clasped hand position too uncomfortable try this alternative which will place less strain on the shoulders. Start the exercise with the hands loosely at your sides. As you go into the forward bend, raise the arms up in a straight line along the sides of the chair and towards the ceiling, still shoulder distance apart (*figure 35*). When you return to the upright position, bring the arms back down to the sides of the chair.

12 Shoulder Opening

FOR: Tension in the shoulder, upper back and neck region.

BENEFITS: Relieves tension in the shoulder, upper back and neck region and increases mobility in the shoulder joints. The stretch works on the sides of the body, the ribs and the armpit area, and opens the chest.

Exercise
1 Sit comfortably with your back, neck and head in a straight line. Place your feet together.
2 Reach for the right shoulder blade with the left hand (*figure 36*). If you cannot reach place the hand in the centre of the upper back. With the right hand hold the left elbow and try to move the elbow gently towards the back of the head. Keep the head and neck in a straight line and look straight ahead whilst doing this. Keep the body centred and do not bend towards the left side. Breathe normally.

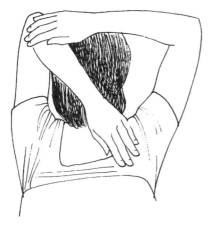

Figure 36

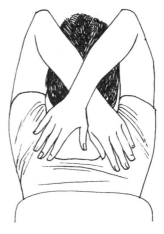

Figure 37

3 After working the shoulder for three to five seconds, release the arms. Rotate the left shoulder to release any tension.
4 Repeat with the right arm.
5 Now try this version with both arms (*figure 37*). It is a little harder, but you can do it. Place the left hand to the right shoulder blade, and the right hand to left shoulder blade. The arms should be crossed behind the head. Keep the head in a straight line and work towards getting both the elbows behind the head, keeping the hands on the shoulders. Hold for three to five seconds and release. Rotate the shoulders to release any tension.

Tip: This is a very hard exercise and many people will experience a lack of mobility in the shoulder joint at first. Persevere and the range of movement will become easier and will increase with practice. It is most important to keep the neck and head straight even if this means you are unable to reach for the shoulder or get the elbow behind the head.

13 Buttock Raising

FOR: Numbness and cramp in the buttocks from prolonged sitting.

BENEFITS: This exercise is a simple movement that can be done throughout the day to ease the tension and increase the circulation in this part of the anatomy. It will also strengthen your arms and shoulders and the thigh muscles.

Exercise
1 Sit towards the front of your chair with your arms holding the seat of the chair slightly behind your body (*figure 38*). The feet should be firmly on the ground, hip-distance apart.
2 Lean backwards, taking the body weight on to the hands, and lift the buttocks off the chair (*figure 39*). Press the weight into the hands to make yourself stable. With the buttocks raised, give the hips a wiggle and sit back down.

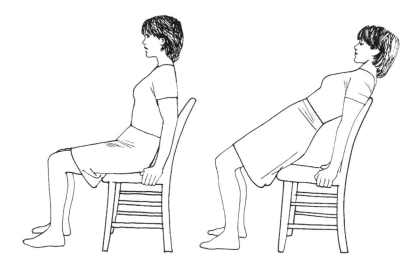

Figure 38   Figure 39

3 Repeat three times.

Tip: Be very careful if your chair has wheels. Keep the feet firmly on the floor to stabilize yourself.

14 Thigh Rocking

FOR: Discomfort, numbness and lack of circulation in the buttock area through sitting for long periods of time.

BENEFITS: Thigh rocking works on all the lower part of your body from the waist downwards. By rocking the thighs, you also release tension from your legs which might be fidgety or stiff from being static for a long period of time. This exercise can be done discreetly throughout the day when you have to sit for prolonged periods of time.

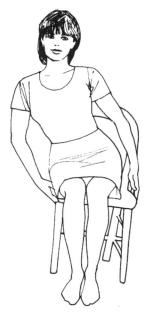

Figure 40

Exercise

1 Place the hands at the back of the seat of the chair.
2 Rock to the right side (*figure 40*), lifting the weight off the left buttock and back to the left side lifting the right buttock off the seat. Rock back and forth for a dozen times.
3 Relax.

Tip: Be very careful not to lean too much to one side as to lose your balance. Hold firmly on to the chair for stability and try and keep both feet on the floor.

15 Leg Bend

FOR: Stiffness of the joints and muscles of the legs.

BENEFITS: Limbers the joints of the leg and stretches the hamstring muscle that runs up the back of the leg, the shin and the heel. In addition it eases indigestion and flatulence.

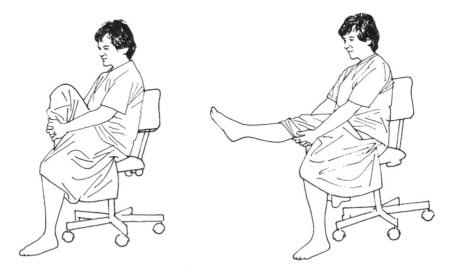

Figure 41   Figure 42

Exercise

1 Sit comfortably with the back, neck and head in a straight line.

2 Lift the right knee to the chest and clasp it with both hands (*figure 41*). Keep the back straight and pull the knee into the chest. Keep the foot relaxed and feel the stomach muscles tighten as the leg is pressed against them. If it helps you can rest the raised foot on the seat of the chair.

3 Stretch the leg out, clasping the hands behind the calf or lower thigh (*figure 42*). If possible, straighten the leg. If this is not possible straighten it as far as you can so you feel the stretch. Keep the back straight using the stomach muscles to hold the body stable.

4 Release and repeat with the left leg.

Tip: An alternative way of doing this exercise is to clasp an old tie or belt around the foot. When you bend the knee to the

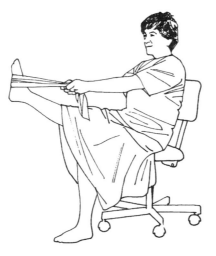

Figure 43

chest, pull on the tie/belt to increase the stretch and straighten the back. When you extend the leg, pull on the belt to feel the resistance and help you to straighten the leg (*figure 43*).

16 Toe and Ankle Exercises

FOR: Stiffness in the toe and ankle joints, poor circulation in the feet and sore and cramped feet due to prolonged standing.

BENEFITS: Stretches the insteps, ankles and tendons of the feet. These simple exercises will increase circulation and will be particularly beneficial to women who wear high heels because the Achilles' tendon is stretched. It is easy to forget the feet when exercising, but the feet take the whole weight of the body and are often crammed into tight shoes for most of the day. It is preferable to do yoga barefoot, but if this is not possible just do your best in your socks or tights.

Exercise
1 Sit straight with the back, neck and head in a straight line. Extend the legs in front of you with the feet resting on the floor.
2 Flex the ankles, so the heels rest on the floor (*figure 44*). Now point the feet so the toes rest on the floor (*figure 45*). Repeat a dozen times. Heels on the floor, toes on the floor.
3 Relax the feet and give them a shake.
4 Now move each foot to the side of the chair. Tuck the toes under and press the front of the foot into the floor (*figure 46*). Feel a stretch up the instep. Hold for three to five seconds, and release.
5 Straighten both legs out in front of you a few inches off the floor. Rotate the feet inwards working the ankle joints for six circles (*figure 47*). Now rotate outwards for six circles.
6 Relax the feet and give them a shake.
7 Finally, extend the legs with the feet raised slightly off the floor. Clench all the toes as tight as possible, and hold for

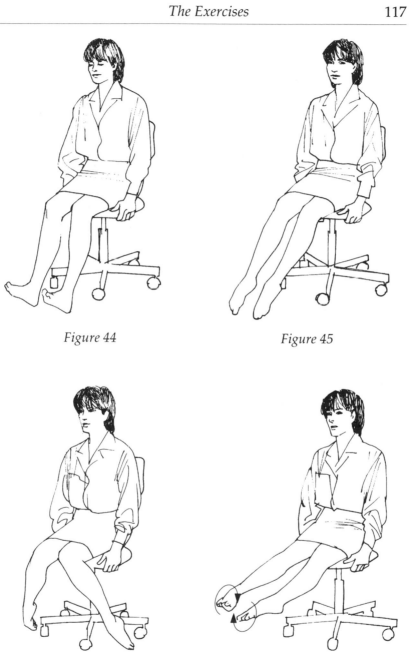

Figure 44

Figure 45

Figure 46

Figure 47

three to five seconds. Now straighten the toes; try to separate them out and feel the air between them. Clench and straighten again three more times.

8 Relax the feet and give them a shake.

Tip: Hold the chair firmly with the hands when raising your feet off the floor. You can do this exercise at intervals during your work without drawing attention to yourself.

17 Knee to Forehead

FOR: Tension and stiffness in the back area.

BENEFITS: Releases tension from the whole back and neck area, eases the joints of the leg and massages the abdomen, releasing any indigestion or flatulence.

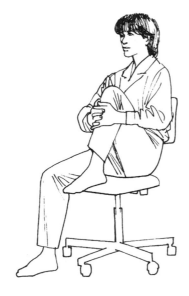
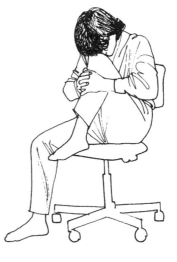

Figure 48a   *Figure 48b*

Exercise

1 Sit with the back, neck and head in a straight line. Clasp the
   knee of the left leg and bring it to the chest (*figure 48a*).
   Exhale, and holding the knee firm to the chest, drop the forehead, chin or nose, towards the knee (*figure 48b*).
2 Hold this stretch for three to five seconds, breathing normally. Feel the stretch up the spine. Do not let the body rock
   backwards, but hold the stomach muscles firm and pull the
   knee into the chest to hold the body stable.
3 Inhale and release the position.
4 Repeat with the right leg.

Tip: Do not do this exercise on a full stomach. The pressure on
your abdomen may cause discomfort or nausea.

18 Eye Exercises

FOR: Sore and strained eyes.

BENEFITS: Strengthens the eye muscles and eases sore and
twitching eyes. If practised regularly, these exercises may help
improve defective vision and delay the need for glasses. We do
not often exercise the eyes, but they are vital organs that are
neglected all too often. Office work can strain the eyes as you
peer at manuscripts, or squint to focus on computer screens. *If
you wear glasses, remove them for this exercise. If you are wearing
contact lenses, you should not attempt this exercise.*

Exercise

1 Sit comfortably with the back, neck and head in a straight line.
2 Stare straight ahead at a spot on the far wall. Keep the gaze
   focused and stare until it becomes uncomfortable. Then close
   your eyes. Repeat three times.
3 Keeping the head still repeat each of these movements five
   times, and close the eyes and relax after each one (*figure 49*).
      i)   Look at the ceiling and then down to the floor.

ii) Look to the right and then to the left.
iii) Look to the upper right corner and to the lower left corner.
iv) Look to the upper left corner and down to the lower right corner.

4 Keeping the head perfectly still, circle the eyes three times to the right and three times to the left. Close the eyes and relax.
5 Rub the palms of the hands quickly together. Now place the cups of the palms over your eyes (*figure 50*). Feel the heat of the palms relax the eyes and their muscles.

Tip: If you feel dizziness or any other discomfort, stop immediately, close your eyes and relax.

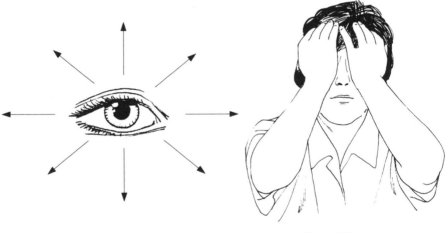

Figure 49   Figure 50

19 Lion Pose

FOR: General tension and lethargy.

BENEFITS: The lion pose is a fun exercise that also has many beneficial effects. The exercise brings extra blood to the facial muscles, tones up your skin, preventing early wrinkles around your eyes and forehead, and is also a superb release of tension. This is not an exercise you will want people to witness, unless they are close friends! Try it at home in front of the mirror.

Exercise
1 Sit comfortably with the back, neck and head in a straight line.
2 Inhale and clench the hands into fists and raise them to the chest.
3 In one movement, exhale the breath from the chest and shoot the hands out, clenching the fingers into claws. At the same time stick the tongue out and open the eyes as wide as possible. Hold the position, let all your tension out through the fingertips, the tongue, the eyes. Feel the heat flood to the face and relax.
4 Repeat one more time – if you have the energy!

Tip: Be careful not to tense the facial muscles too hard. Only hold the position for two to five seconds.

20 Temple, Face and Head Massage

FOR: Tension in the head and facial muscles.

BENEFITS: The face often mirrors how we feel. When we feel stressed, the facial muscles will be tense, and when we are happy they will be relaxed. A simple self-massage of the temple, face and head can go a long way to ease tension. By massaging the pressure points, it is possible to ease headaches and sinus pain and to leave yourself feeling relaxed and calm. The jaw, in particular, accumulates a lot of tension, and it is important to release this through simple movements of the mouth.

Remember to be very gentle and to apply only a light pressure when carrying out the massage movements. Be particularly careful if you have long fingernails. We indicate below which fingers to use, but this is only for guidance, and you can adapt it as necessary.

Exercise

1 Sit comfortably. Using the first three fingers of each hand massage the temples in a small circular motion (*figure 51a*). Be gentle and do not press too hard.

2 Now using the tips of all your fingers and thumbs in a small, circular motion, massage the forehead for six times (*figure 51b*).

3 Using the balls of the fingers massage around the eyes, very gently for three circles (*figure 51c*).

4 With the middle fingers massage between the eyebrows in very small circular movements.

5 Now run the first and second fingers from the bridge of the nose down across the cheek bones, pressing gently (*figure 51d*).

6 Massage the upper lip and the area at the side of the nose.

7 With all the fingers massage around the mouth and the chin, feeling how the lower jaw is loose and relaxed (*figure 51e*).

8 Move the jaw from side to side and make yawning movements.

9 Now place the thumbs at the base of the skull. Cradle the head with the hands and slowly massage the base of the skull with the thumbs (*figure 51f*).

10 Gently massage your scalp with your fingers.

Tip: Be very careful if you have long nails or are wearing jewellery. If you are wearing makeup at work, you may prefer to leave this exercise for home.

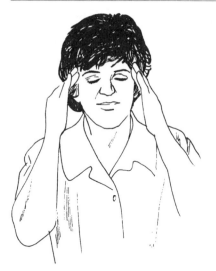

Figure 51a

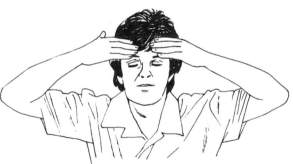

Figure 51b

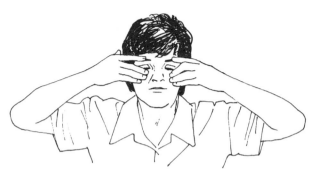

Figure 51c

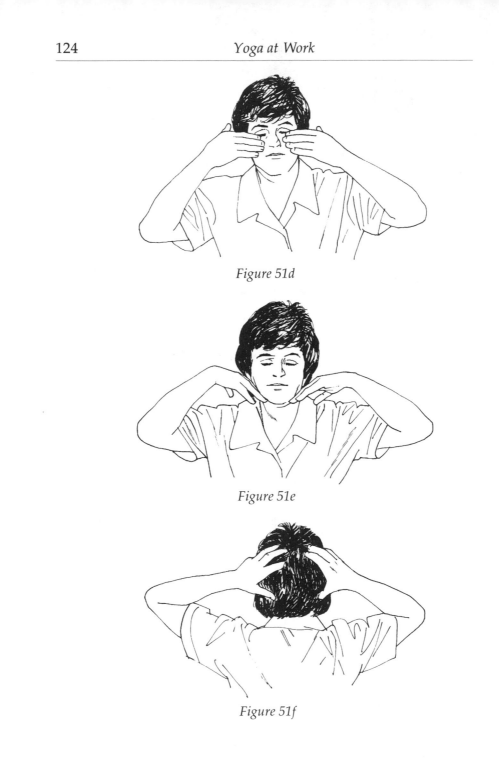

Figure 51d

Figure 51e

Figure 51f

21 Free Stretch

FOR: Unwanted tension in the body.

BENEFITS: This stretch releases the body of tension and stiffness. It mobilizes the whole body and leaves you feeling refreshed.

Exercise
This exercise can be done sitting down, standing or even lying on the floor. The purpose of the exercise is to listen to the body and to stretch in whatever way and direction you want. There is no right or wrong way; just do whatever feels good! Stretch the arms, the legs, the fingers, the toes, the back, the sides, the face muscles and anything else you can think of. Make the movements fluid and overcome any stiffness or slight discomfort by imagining yourself as supple and loose. Imagine you are dancing, or bathed in warm sunlight. Some people find it helpful to think of a cat, stretching its body in long luxurious movements.

Tip: Remove your tie and loosen your collar before you do this stretch. The looser your clothes the more freedom of movement you will have.

STANDING EXERCISES

1 Squatting

FOR: Stiff joints, poor circulation and general feeling of lethargy.

BENEFITS: Loosens up the ankles and knees, and increases the circulation in the whole body. This exercise also strengthens the leg muscles, in particular those of the thighs and bottom. The movement will also strengthen the abdomen muscles and improve your balance. Squatting is particularly beneficial after sitting for long periods of time.

Exercise

1 Stand up with the feet hip-distance apart and hold the back of your chair, or the side of your desk (*figure 52*).
2 Drop the body into a squatting position; take the body weight on your toes with the heels off the floor (*figure 53*). Keep the back straight and look ahead.
3 Using your stomach muscles, raise the body to the standing position with heels flat on the floor.
4 Repeat this movement five to ten times, increasing the speed.
5 Relax and shake out your legs.

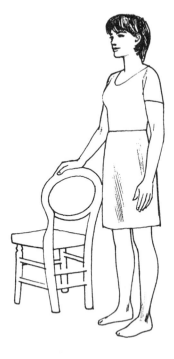

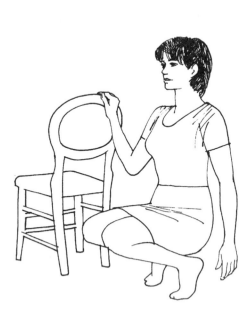

Figure 52   *Figure 53*

Tip: Do not worry if this exercise makes your joints click; this is usually just a sign that your body is beginning to move again! If, however, this is accompanied by any pain, you should stop immediately.

2 Rib Opening

FOR: Stiff, cramped muscles and general lethargy.

BENEFITS: Stretches the whole side of your body from your hip, waist, ribs and shoulders right through to your armpit, arm and hand. When you get up in the morning, you give the body a stretch to get the joints back into action, increase the circulation and generally wake up the body. Similarly, after you have been sitting still for a long time, the body will benefit from a good stretch.

Exercise
1 Standing straight with the feet together, raise the hands above the head, shoulder distance apart.
2 Reach for the ceiling with each hand alternately. As you do so, feel the whole side of the body stretch; your waist, your ribs front and back and the shoulder, arm and hand (*figure 54* over the page). Feel with each stretch that you are becoming two inches taller on that side.
3 Repeat for five to ten times, and relax.

Tip: Tight clothing might restrict your movement. Loosen your tie and collar, and remove your jacket for this exercise.

3 Forward Bend with Chest Expansion

FOR: Stiffness in the back and shoulders, and hamstring and breathing problems.

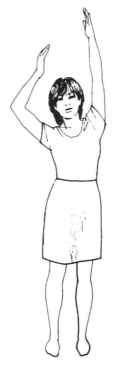

Figure 54

BENEFITS: Opens the whole chest area, stretches the back and hamstrings. This exercise combines the all-important forward bend with chest expansion. It is a wonderful stretch for your back, upper arms, shoulders and shoulder blades. The forward bend movement also massages the stomach muscles and can bring comfort from digestive problems.

Exercise

1 Stand straight with your feet hip-distance apart and the hands clasped behind the back (*figure 55*).
2 Inhale. Exhale and bend the body forward, keeping the legs straight. As you bend the arms will rise behind the back, still with hands clasped (*figure 56*). Keep the head slightly up

until you have completed half of the movement and then let it hang naturally.

3 Hold this position for three to five seconds, breathing normally. Remember to keep the shoulders open, the arms and the legs as straight as possible. Feel the pull of gravity make the body become heavy and lower with each breath.

4 When you have had enough, slowly roll up the spine with the head coming up last, lowering the arms as you do so. Release the arms and relax.

Tip: As with all the forward bend movements, take particular care if you suffer from high blood pressure. If you keep the eyes open throughout this exercise, it will reduce the risk of dizziness when you return to the upright position.

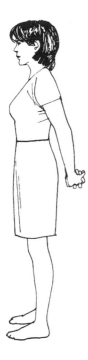

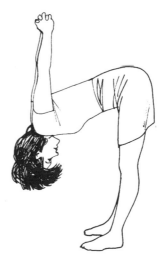

Figure 55   *Figure 56*

4 Forward Bend

FOR: Stiffness in the spine and hamstrings.

BENEFITS: Increases flexibility of the spine. The forward bend
has many benefits: it will release tension from the back region,
stretch the backs of the legs and increase the suppleness of the
spine. The forward bend also brings the blood to the head and
so nourishes the facial muscles and the brain cells. The internal
organs will also be massaged as the bend puts pressure on the
abdominal region.

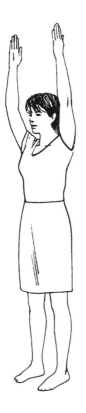

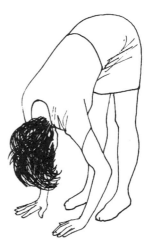

Figure 57   *Figure 58*

Exercise

1 Stand straight with your feet slightly apart. Lift the arms above the head, shoulder-distance apart (*figure 57*). Inhale and reach towards the ceiling.

2 Breathe out and, feeling that the base of the spine is reaching for the ceiling and the arms are reaching towards the floor, bend forwards as far as you can (*figure 58*). Just let the body hang, feeling the gravity pull you nearer to the floor. The head should be between the arms, looking towards your legs. The arms should be relaxed and dropping towards the floor. If you are very supple, you may be able to put your hands flat on the floor.

3 Hold this position for three to five seconds, breathing normally. Feel the tip of the spine reaching for the ceiling and your chest reaching towards the floor. Keep the eyes open. Try and keep the heels on the floor and the backs of the legs straight. It is better to keep the legs straight and to not lower the back so far. If it is more comfortable, you can hold onto your legs to give you stability.

4 When you are ready, slowly begin to roll up the spine. Keep the arms at the side of the head as you do this. Roll up from the bottom of the spine with the head returning to position last.

5 Do the backwards bend (see p. 132) as the counter pose.

Tip: If you suffer from high blood pressure or dizziness, be particularly careful when doing this exercise. If you feel any dizziness or ringing in the ears, return to the standing position immediately. Remember to stretch only as far as feels comfortable; do not over-extend your body. It is very important to keep the legs straight, and it will be more beneficial to maintain this and not to bend forward so far.

5 Backwards Bend

FOR: Stiffness and tension in the back region.

BENEFITS: Increases the flexibility of the spine and eases tension in the back region. After the forwards bend, you should always do the backwards bend as the counter stretch. This stretch also releases tension in the back, increases the flexibility of the spine and opens the chest region.

Exercise
1 Standing straight with your legs hip-distance apart, place the hands on the buttocks or the waist for support. If you prefer you can hold the back of a chair for support. Keep the eyes open throughout this exercise.

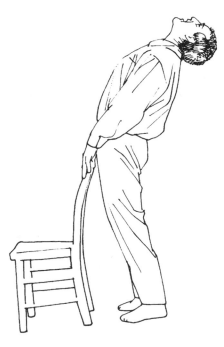

Figure 59

2 Inhale. Exhale, and with the knees slightly bent for stability bend slightly backwards (*figure 59*). Only go as far as is comfortable and so you can feel a gentle stretch of the back. Do not drop the head backwards if this feels uncomfortable, but keep it in line with the chest with the face towards the ceiling.

3 Hold this position for three to five seconds, breathing normally. You may feel a slight restriction of the breath, but this is natural.

4 Inhale and slowly roll up and return to the upright position.

Tip: If you prefer, you can hold on to the edge of a chair or desk with one hand for support during the backwards bend. Remember to be particularly careful with the position of the head. Only lift the face gently towards the ceiling, do not jar the neck by dropping the head backwards. Keep the eyes open during this exercise, to prevent any dizziness.

6 The Spinal Twist

FOR: Stiffness and tension in the back and hips.

BENEFITS: Increases flexibility of the spine and tones the abdominal area. This is a variation on the sitting spinal twist. The twist movement brings pressure on your internal organs and works on your kidney, spleen, liver and adrenal glands. It increases the suppleness of the spine and improves the condition of the spinal vertebrae. If done correctly the spinal twist also opens the chest and shoulder area and improves posture.

Exercise
1 Stand with the feet together, and interlock the hands behind your head. Keep the elbows open and do not pull on the head.

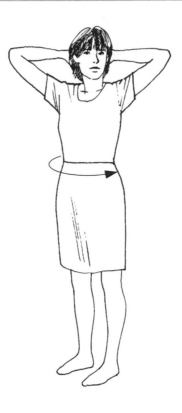

Figure 60

2 Keeping the hips facing the front, twist to the right wall and
   then to the left wall (*figure 60*). Twist three times to each side.
   Try to keep your elbows open as you do so.
3 Relax.

Tip: In order to feel the full benefit of the stretch it is important
to keep the hips facing the front and just move the body from
the waist upwards as you twist. Remember to keep the elbows
open so that you are keeping the chest open.

7 Triangle

FOR: Stiffness and tension in the back, ribs and waist area.

BENEFITS: Improves flexibility and condition of the spine and tones the waistline. This is a classical hatha yoga exercise. The triangle movement keeps the spine flexible, tones up your waistline and will bring blood to your head. Again, the bending movement will massage the internal organs. The position of the feet may take a little time to master, but it will soon become familiar.

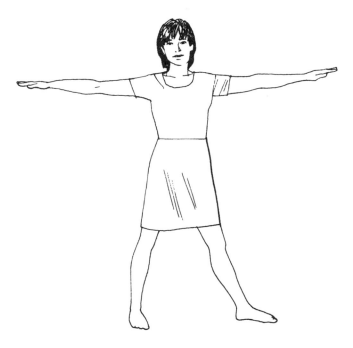

Figure 61

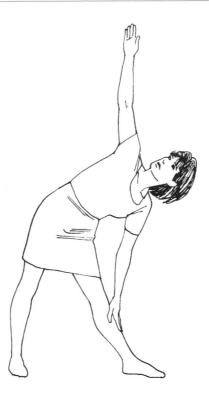

Figure 62

Exercise

1 Stand with the feet about 2–3 feet apart and the body facing forwards. Turn the left foot in to a 45° angle. Turn the right foot out to a 90° angle. Keep the hips facing the front (*figure 61*).

2 Now raise the arms to shoulder level at the sides of the body. Inhale. Exhale and reaching out with the right hand, bend the body to the left. The left hand will reach for the floor, or if more comfortable rest it on your foot or shin. The right hand will reach for the ceiling. In the classical yoga positions, the face should be turned towards the raised hand. If you find this uncomfortable, keep the head in line with the chest and face forwards. (*figure 62*).

3 Hold this position for three to five seconds, breathing normally. Rest the left hand on the knee, shin or even the foot for support. Try to keep the legs straight and to feel an opening of the chest.
4 Inhale and slowly return to the upright position.
5 Repeat this stretch to the right side. This time the right foot will be turned in at a 45° angle and the left foot will be turned out at a 90° angle.

Tip: Be careful with the position of your head. If you feel any discomfort keep it in line with the shoulders and the chest.

8 The Dancer Balance

FOR: Lack of concentration.

BENEFITS: Focusing the mind, stretching the front of the thigh and hip region. Balance is an important aspect of yoga; to balance is to master and control the body and mind. It results in confidence, increased concentration, grace, poise and steadiness of the mind. The dancer balance also stretches the thigh of the raised leg and works on the pelvic area.
    To balance successfully in a certain position, you have to focus the eyes on a particular spot and concentrate. It requires a positive attitude; say to yourself 'I will not wobble and lose my balance'. Try this simple exercise, but do not be disheartened if you find it hard at first.

Exercise
1 Stand with your feet together. Extend the right arm at the side of the head, with the tips of the fingers reaching for the ceiling. With the left hand, reach for the left foot and pull it into the left buttock (*figure 63*).
2 Hold this position for three to five seconds, breathing normally. Focus on a spot in front of you to help you balance. Feel the stretch up the left thigh as you pull the foot into the

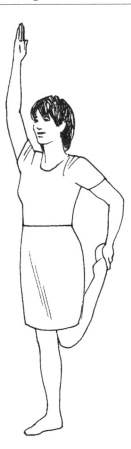

Figure 63

buttock. Feel the stretch up the right side as the arm reaches
towards the ceiling. Release the foot and return to the normal
standing position.
3 Repeat with the left arm reaching for the ceiling and the right
foot to the right buttock.

Tip: Do not worry if you cannot hold this balance for very long
at first – this is perfectly natural! If it helps, hold on to a wall for
support until your balance improves.

9 Variation on the Cat Pose

FOR: Stiffness and tension in the back and chest area.

BENEFITS: Works on the flexibility of the spine, and eases backache and other tension in this region. This exercise is called the cat pose because it resembles a cat when it stretches. It mobilizes the spine and the muscles of the back region, massages the lumbar region and is very beneficial for people with back problems.

Exercise
1 Stand with your hands holding the back of a chair or the edge of a desk. Take a big step backwards so you are able to flatten the back with the feet slightly apart and the hands the same distance apart holding the desk/chair (*figure 64*). The legs should be straight, the chest should be reaching for the floor and the head should be between the arms facing the floor too.
2 In this position, lift the head up and arch the back (*figure 65*). Feel this stretch the whole length of the spine.
3 Now reverse the position; look down to the ground and hump the back (*figure 66*). Again, feel this stretch. Repeat this

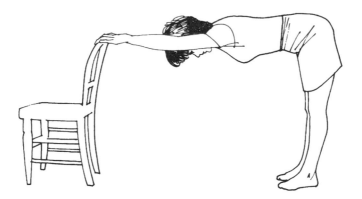

Figure 64

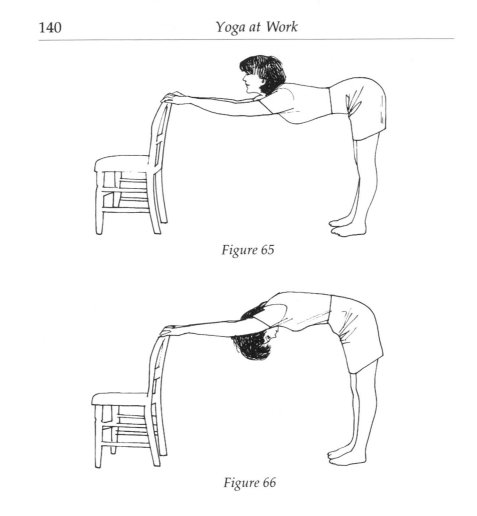

Figure 65

Figure 66

movement, arch with the feet flat and hump your back while on the tip of the toes, three times. Wiggle the back and hips to relax.

Tip: Take care not to strain the neck by moving the head too vigorously. Just let the head follow the movement of the back.

13

Practice Programmes

We recommend that you try and do ten to fifteen minutes of yoga a day at work. These practice programmes are designed to help you structure your yoga practice and ensure you get a balanced workout. There are five suggested programmes, each including breathing, a selection of exercises and relaxation.

When you are familiar with the exercises, you might prefer to make up your own programme, tailored to your specific needs and the amount of time you have to spare. Always start with a few breathing exercises. These will get you in the right frame of mind. Do the full breath exercise, and add some of the basic breathing exercises each day. Then choose five or six exercises from the sitting exercises, and at least two from the standing exercises. If your time is limited, try to do at least five minutes of breathing and five minutes of relaxation – it will be time well spent! If you have more time, try to do as many of the exercises as you can.

Do not be rigid with your practice programmes, try and vary them as much as possible and adapt them to meet your needs. Do not worry if you occasionally miss a day's yoga practice. If you do, try and do a few exercises at home. We have not included going for a walk in the above programme, but we presume you will do so, weather permitting, in order to get some fresh air.

Suggested programmes

Programme 1	Exercise	Page	Main benefits	Time
Whole body workout	1 Breathing	75	1 Calms and focuses the mind and body	3–5 mins
	2 Neck and head roll	89	2 Eases tension and stiffness in the neck, shoulder and upper back region	30 secs–1 min
	3 Fingers and wrists	96	3 Eases stiffness and tenderness in the fingers and wrists from repetitive movements	1 min
	4 Forward bend (standing)	130	4 Improves flexibility and condition of the spine, stretches the hamstrings, brings blood to the face	30 secs–1 min
	5 Triangle (standing)	135	5 Improves flexibility of the spine and the hamstrings and tones the whole body	1 min
	6 Rib opening	127	6 Provides an overall body stretch which energizes and refreshes the body	1 min
	7 Relaxation	84	7 Calms and focuses the mind, releases the body from all unwanted tension and leaves you feeling refreshed and serene	3–5 mins **Total** 10–15 mins

Programme 2	Exercise	Page	Main benefits	Time
Whole body workout	1 Breathing	75	1 Calms and focuses the mind and body	3–5 mins
	2 Shoulder lifts and rotation	91	2 Eases tension in the shoulder and upper back area	30 secs–1 min
	3 Shoulder and arm rotation	93	3 Increases mobility of the shoulder blades	30 secs–1 min
	4 Spinal twist	107	4 Increases the flexibility of the spine and tones the abdomen	1 min
	5 Triangle (standing)	135	5 Increases the flexibility of the spine and stretches and tones the waist area	1 min
	6 Forward bend with chest	127	6 Increases the flexibility of the spine, stretches the hamstrings, opens the chest and upper back area	1 min
	7 Relaxation	84	7 Calms and focuses the mind, releases the body from all unwanted tension and leaves you feeling refreshed and serene	3–5 mins **Total** 10–15 mins

Programme 3	Exercise	Page	Main benefits	Time
All sitting workout	1 Breathing	75	1 Calms and focuses the mind and body	3–5 mins
	2 Arm stretch	93	2 Stretches the arm muscles and tendons	1 min
	3 Shoulder opening	110	3 Mobilizes the shoulder blades	1 min
	4 Buttock raising	112	4 Eases feelings of numbness and cramp in the buttock area	1 min
	5 Thigh rocking	113	5 Brings circulation back to the buttock area	1 min
	6 Toes and ankles	116	6 Eases stiffness in the toes and ankles, increases circulation to the lower legs	1 min
	7 Leg bend	114	7 Stretches the hamstrings	1 min
	8 Relaxation	84	8 Calms and focuses the mind, releases the body from all unwanted tension and leaves you feeling refreshed and serene	5 mins
				Total 14–16 mins

Programme 4	Exercise	Page	Main benefits	Time
Whole body workout	1 Breathing	75	1 Calms and focuses the mind and body	3–5 mins
	2 Arm stretch	93	2 Stretches the arm muscles and tendons	30 secs–1 min
	3 Knee to forehead	118	3 Increases the flexibility of the spine, massages the abdomen	30 secs–1 min
	4 Eye exercises	119	4 Exercises the eye muscles, soothes eye strain	1 min
	5 Lion pose	120	5 Releases general tension	30 secs–1 min
	6 Forward bend with chest expansion (standing)	127	6 Increases the flexibility of the spine, stretches the hamstrings, opens the chest and upper back area	30 secs–1 min
	7 Cat pose	139	7 Eases tension in the whole back	1 min
	8 Relaxation	84	8 Calms and focuses the mind, releases the body from all unwanted tension and leaves you feeling refreshed and serene	3–5 mins
				Total 10–16 mins

Programme 5	Exercise	Page	Main benefits	Time
All standing workout	1 Breathing	75	1 Calms and focuses the mind and body	3–5 mins
	2 Squatting	125	2 Mobilizes the joints	1 min
	3 Rib opening	127	3 An overall body stretch which energizes the body	30 secs–1 min
	4 Forward bend (standing)	130	4 Improves the flexibility and condition of the spine, stretches the hamstrings, brings blood to the face	30 secs–1 min
	5 Back bend (standing)	132	5 Increases flexibility of the spine, eases tension in the back	30 secs–1 min
	6 Triangle (standing)	135	6 Increases flexibility of the spine, tones the abdomen, opens the chest and shoulder region, stretches the hamstrings	1 min
	7 Spinal twist (standing)	133	7 Increases flexibility of the spine, tones the waist area	30 secs–1 min
	8 Cat pose	139	8 Eases tension in the whole back	1 min
	9 Dancer balance	137	9 Increases concentration and poise	1 min
	10 Relaxation/meditation	84/86	10 Calms and focuses the mind, releases the body from all unwanted tension and leaves you feeling refreshed and serene	3–5 mins
				Total 12–18 mins

Conclusion

By reading this book you have probably already begun to think more about stress in your work life, identified potential causes and observed how it affects you. Hopefully you have also begun to think more positively about how you can make small changes that will improve your well-being at work. These may include trying to adopt a more positive attitude, listening to your body and practising yoga at work. We cannot offer solutions in this book, but hopefully we can set you on the right path and encourage thought processes that will enable you to address your personal problem areas with a renewed spirit.

Work takes up much of our time and is undoubtedly an important part of our lives, but it should not have a negative effect on our time away from the workplace. If you feel drained of energy, unhappy or even ill at the end of the working day, something is wrong; do not accept that you have to feel like this! We hope that you will now be able to explore and identify the causes of any stress problems and take some positive action towards alleviating them.

We must not, of course, forget the yoga exercises which are the focus of this book. We firmly believe that yoga can greatly enhance your working life; it can counter physical and mental problems, equip you better to cope with stress in general and can make you feel more relaxed and content at work. But this does not happen without regular practice and perseverance. Your body is a most precious resource, one that has to last your whole life; invest a little time in looking after it at work. Your perseverance will be rewarded by a sense of well-being which, as Dr Chandra states in his foreword, will then become the incentive for continuation.

Whether young, old or too old, sick or lean, one who discards laziness gets success if he practises yoga.
Success comes to him who is engaged in the practice; for by merely reading books on yoga, one can never get success.
Success cannot be attained by adopting a particular dress.
It cannot be gained by telling tales.
Practice alone is the means of success.

Hatha Yoga Pradipika

The Philosophy of Yoga

It is not necessary to know the history of yoga to develop and progress in hatha yoga. But for those who wish to pursue the study of yoga before reading further books or joining a class, it might be helpful to know how it originated and developed. Hatha yoga is a self-developmental system; it focuses on the physical, emotional, mental and spiritual aspects of our life. Yoga means union; union of the physical and spiritual part of man.

Patanjali is considered to be the father of yoga. He lived in India in approximately 300BC, and wrote the yoga sutras or aphorisms, which number approximately 196. This work is divided into four parts: the aim of yoga; the practice of yoga; power; liberation. Patanjali advocates the eight steps of yoga, sometimes referred to as the ladder of yoga, and these consist of:

1 Yamas (practices from which we should abstain)
2 Niyamas (practices which we should observe)
3 Posture
4 Breathing
5 Sense of withdrawal
6 Concentration
7 Meditation
8 High state of consciousness or super-consciousness

The philosophy of yoga sets out high ethics for daily living. Patanjali's yamas and niyamas provide guidelines for what to abstain from and what to observe on a daily basis:

To abstain	To observe
1 Not to harm anything	1 Purity
2 To be honest	2 Contentedness
3 Not to steal	3 Restraint
4 Moral conduct	4 Study
5 Not to be greedy	5 Devotion

If, through our daily living, we remember and practise these ten principles of Patanjali, we will definitely progress in yoga.

Posture, breathing and meditation are dealt with it in this book. Sense of withdrawal (No 5) refers to detaching oneself from the external stimuli of our lives and focusing within ourselves. This state will be the starting point for Concentration (No 6) and the subsequent two states of meditation and super-consciousness.

Patanjali does not refer to the yoga postures in great detail in his writing. He only mentions the need for a steady posture for meditation. *The Hatha Yoga Pradipika, Siva Samhita* and *Gheranda Samhita* are considered the authorities on hatha yoga, but these three texts are only for serious students of the subject.

Most yoga classes combine hatha yoga (the physical exercises) with raja yoga (the mental exercises) as we cannot separate the body and the mind. Raja yoga, sometimes also referred to as the royal path, teaches us how to control the mind and to still it. There are a number of methods to achieve this which include effort, the right attitude and non-attachment. Non-attachment in basic terms means that we should not be overly attached to material goods or even people. Of course this is very difficult to achieve in today's society, and worldly things do have a place, but they should not be the focus of our life. We should not be so attached to material things that if we lose them we are devastated. If we lost them all we would still have ourselves and so to a certain extent would still be 'rich'. Happiness should come from within and not be reliant on possessions, relationships and other external stimuli. This is the message of non-attachment.

Yoga is referred to in the Hindu scriptures, *The Upanishads,* which were written around 1,000BC, and *The Bhagavad Gita*, written around 300BC. *The Upanishads* refer to the idea of one God, the supreme being, and establish the teacher/disciple relationship; the idea that everyone travelling the yoga path should have a master, someone who can guide you on your journey because they too have travelled the path before. *The Bhagavad Gita* provides a guide for anyone travelling the yoga path which ultimately leads to man uniting himself with the supreme being.

Yoga was introduced to the West by a succession of teachers from the East. Of particular note is B K S Iyengar, who during the 1950s increased the popularity of yoga by introducing evening yoga classes. Today there are a number of systems of yoga in existence, many following the teaching of a particular person or school of yoga, for example, Iyengar, Sivananda and Gitananda.

In addition to the spiritual guidance, yoga philosophy also provides guidance on keeping the body healthy, via the yoga postures and diet and cleanliness. The physical yoga exercises have a number of benefits which we refer to in the earlier chapters 'What is Yoga?' and 'How Yoga Can Help'. Yoga is now taken seriously by the medical profession as it has been found through research that yoga exercises, and the breathing and relaxation techniques in particular, can help a number of ailments. Examples include asthma, cardio-vascular conditions and high blood pressure.

Further Reading

There is a large range of books available on the topics covered by this book. Below is a selection which the authors have found particularly useful.

Yoga Philosophy
Bernard, T, *Hatha Yoga*, Rider & Co, 1976.
Gandhi, M K, *The Bhagavad Gita*, Orient Paperbacks, 1971.
Iyengar, B K S, *Light on Yoga*, Thorsons, 1966.
Nath, I, *Yoga, The Classical Way*, Patanjali Yoga Centre.
Satyananda, *Asana, Pranayam, Mudra, Bandha*, Bihar School of Yoga, 1969.
Sivananda, *Health and Hatha Yoga*, Sivananda Group.
Swami Prabhavananda & Isherwood, A, *How to Know God: The Yoga Aphorisms of Patanjali*, Mentor Book, New American Library Inc, 1969.
Swami Prabhavananda & Manchester, F, (translators), *The Upanishads*, Vedanta Press, 1983.
Vishnudevandanda, *The Hatha Yoga Pradapika*, Om Lotus Publications, 1987.
Vivekananda, *Raja Yoga*, Advaita Ashrama, 1994.

General Yoga
Balaskas, J, *Preparing for Birth with Yoga*, Element Books, 1994.
Berg, V, *Yoga for Pregnancy*, Watkins, 1981 (currently out of print).
Devereux, G, *The Elements of Yoga*, Element Books, 1994.
Hewitt, J, *Teach Yourself Yoga*, Teach Yourself Publications, 1992.
Hittleman, *28-Day Exercise Plan*, Bantam Books, 1971.
Kent, H, *The Complete Yoga Course*, Headline, 1994.

Phelan, *Yoga for Women*, Arrow Books, 1979.
Sivananda Group, *Learn Yoga in a Weekend*, Ebury Press, 1994.
Svami Purna, *Balanced Yoga*, Element Books, 1993.
Vishnudevananda, *The Complete Book of Yoga*, Sivananda Group.
Yesudian & Haich, *Yoga Week-by-Week*, Thorsons, 1976.

Relaxation & Meditation
Chaitow, L, *Relaxation & Meditation Techniques*, Thorsons, 1984.
Hambly, K., *Overcoming Tension*, Sheldon Press, 1983.
Hewitt, J, *Teach Yourself Meditation*, Teach Yourself Publications, 1984.
Humphreys, C, *Concentration and Meditation*, Element Books, 1993.
Le Shan, L, *How to Meditate*, Aquarian, 1993.
Ram Dass, *Journey of Awakening*, Bantam Books, 1978.
Yogaswami, *Positive Thoughts for Daily Meditation*, Element Books, 1993.

Inspiration & Spiritual Growth
Bach, R, *Jonathan Livingston Seagull*, Turnstone Press, 1972.
Freedman, M, *Under the Mango Tree*, Astoria Publications, 1989.
Gilbran, K, *The Prophet*, Pan Books, 1991.
Scott Peck, M, *Further Along the Road Less Travelled*, Simon & Schuster, 1994.
Shah, I, *Learning How to Learn*, Penguin, 1983.
Tweedie, I, *The Chasm of Fire*, Element Books, 1993.

Most of the books on this list are available by mail order from Angela's Books & Tapes, 7 St Nicholas Crescent, Banchory, Kincardineshire, Scotland, AB31 3YF, telephone +44 (01330) 823317.

Useful Addresses

Australia
International Yoga Teachers'
 Association
c/o 14/15 Huddart Avenue
Normanhurst
NSW 2076

Canada
Sivananda Yoga Vedanta Centre
5178 St Lawrence Blvd
Montreal
QUE H2T 1R8

Sivananda Yoga Vedanta Centre
77 Harbord Street
Toronto
ONT M5S 1G4

Unity in Yoga
303 2495 W2nd Avenue
Vancouver
BC VGK 1J5

Israel
Israeli Yoga Teachers'
 Association
c/o PO Box 48087
Tel Aviv 61480

Sivananda Yoga Vedanta Centre
11 Ein Ha Kareh
Tel Aviv 66028

New Zealand
Eswaran & Kalyan Balzer
70 Callipe Road
Devanport
Auckland

South Africa
Anada Kutir Yoga Centre
24 Sprigg Road
Rondesbosch East 7780
Cape Town

Renuka Mandan
136 Prince Edward Street
Flat 3, Himal Court
Durban 4001
Natal

United Kingdom
British Wheel of Yoga
1 Hamilton Place
Boston Road
Sleaford
Lincs NG34 7ES

Iyengar Yoga Centre
223A Randolf Avenue
Maida Vale
London W9 1NL

Patanjali Yoga Centre & Ashram
The Cott
Marley Lane
Battle
Sussex TN33 0RE

Sivananda Yoga Vedanta Centre
51 Felsham Road
London SW15 1AZ

United States
Sivananda Yoga Vedanta Center
243 West 24th Street
New York NY 10011

Unity in Yoga International
PO Box 281004
Lakewood
Colorado 80228

Unity Yoga International
7918 Bolling Drive
Alexandria
Virginia 22308

Yogaville
Buckingham
Virginia 23921

Contemplative Thoughts

To dream of the person you would like to be
is to waste the person you are.

Anonymous

Sometime you wonder how you got on this mountain.
But sometimes you wonder, how will I get off.

Joan Manley

Those who lose dreaming are lost.

Australian Aboriginal Proverb

There are two kinds of people, those who do
the work and those who take the credit. Try to be
in the first group; there is less competition there.

Indira Gandhi

A loving heart is the truest wisdom.

Charles Dickens

The greatest power is often simple patience.

E Joseph Cossman

If you imagine it, you can achieve it, if you
can dream it, you can become it.

William Arthur Ward

Better keep yourself clean and bright;
you are the window through which you
must see the world.

George Bernard Shaw

The wise have inherited wisdom by means
of silence and contemplation.

Meshadel Dinowouri

No door leads
to happiness or unhappiness.
Both enter in when you ask them to.

Japanese Wisdom

Even the thousand mile road has a first step.

Japanese Wisdom

Serenity is neither frivolity, nor complacency,
it is the highest knowledge and love,
it is the affirmation of all reality being awake
at the edge of all deeps and abysses

Serenity is the secret of beauty
and the real substance of art.

Hermann Hesse

What is the use of love,
good fortune,
knowledge and riches,
if you do not give
yourself time
to enjoy them in leisure?

Gleichen Russwurm

One who is at peace and is quiet
no sorrow or harm can enter,
no evil breath can invade.
Therefore his inner power
remains whole and his spirit intact.

Chuang Tzu

Who is wise?
The man who can learn something from everyone.
Who is strong?
The man who overcomes his passion.
Who is rich?
The man who is content with his fate.
Whom do men honor?
The man who honors his fellow man.

Sayings of the Fathers

Condemn no man
and consider nothing impossible,

for there is no man who does not have
a future,
and there is nothing that does not
have its hour.

The Talmud

The supreme happiness of life
is the conviction that we are loved.

Victor Hugo

An hour of concentrated work does
more to kindle joy, to overcome sadness
and to set your ship afloat again, than a
month of gloomy brooding.

Benjamin Franklin

Seek not to have that everything should be
as you wish, but wish for everything to
happen as it actually does happen and
you will be serene.

Epictetus

As you move on the pathway of life,
do not look for obstacles, difficulties,
dangers.
Look only for opportunities.

J P Vaswani

In the midst of your daily work, in the
tumult and storm of life, pause for a while,
again and again.

J P Vaswani

I do my thing, and you do your thing.
I am not in this world to live up to your
expectations.
And you are not in this world to live
up to mine.
You are you and I am I,
And if by chance we find each other,
its beautiful.
If not, it can't be helped.

Frederick S Perl
Gestalt Therapy Prayer

What the world really needs
is more love and less paperwork.

Pearl Bailey

Meditation is not a means to
an end. It is both the means and
the end.

Krishna Murthi

To meditate is to be innocent
of time.

Krishna Murthi

Meditation is the action of silence.

Krishna Murthi

We don't make mistakes
We just have learnings.

Anne Wilson-Schaef

Not many of us realize the value of laughter.
Laughter is both physical and spiritual tonic.
We should, however, be careful to see that
we do not laugh at others. Let us laugh
with others and let us laugh at ourselves.

J P Vaswami

Index